Seated Tai Chi for Seniors Over 60

A Fully Illustrated 28-Day Chair Exercise Plan for Better Balance,
Stronger Joints, and Sharper Mind — Just 10 Minutes Daily

Liuhe Chen

Disclaimer

The content in this book is provided for educational purposes and general guidance only. Nothing here replaces a consultation with your doctor or a qualified medical professional. Before starting this seated program or any new form of physical activity, please speak with your physician, especially if you are managing a chronic condition, recovering from injury or surgery, or have recently been unwell.

The author and publisher have taken care to present this material responsibly. Even so, neither accepts liability for any adverse outcome, injury, or loss that may arise from following the guidance in these pages. Use your own judgment, listen to your body, and consult a professional when in doubt.

Table of Contents

A Note from the Author

My grandmother practiced Tai Chi every morning until she was eighty-three. She had a small garden and a wooden stool she moved to different corners depending on the light. She was not doing anything dramatic. She lifted her arms, shifted her weight side to side, breathed through movements that looked almost like nothing from the outside. But her hands never shook. Her mind stayed sharp. She moved through her days with a steadiness that had nothing to do with not being old. It had to do with never stopping.

I thought about her when I started working with older adults who had given up on exercise. Not given up because they were unwilling. Given up because the options they had been offered did not fit the bodies they were living in. Stand on one leg. Walk on a treadmill. Use the gym equipment. These instructions were given without unkindness, but they were given to the wrong body at the wrong time.

What those people needed was not a modified version of something else. They needed something built for them from the start. A program where the chair is the foundation, not the fallback.

That is what this book is.

The ten exercises you will learn here are drawn from the same slow-movement principles that have kept bodies like my grandmother's functional and mobile into old age. The difference is that every exercise in this program is done from a chair. Not because I am lowering the bar. Because the chair creates specific conditions that make certain kinds of training more precise, more accessible, and more sustainable than their standing equivalents.

When you sit in a stable chair, you do not have to spend energy managing a standing balance demand at the same time as doing something deliberate with your arms and trunk. That freed attention goes somewhere. It goes into the quality of the movement, into the breath, into the kind of slow, purposeful joint work that actually changes how a stiff shoulder feels in the morning or how far you can reach across a table without bracing yourself.

The three things this program is designed to improve are the three things I have heard the same people mention over and over again across many years of this work. They want to feel less wobbly. They want their joints to stop complaining every time they move. And they want their thinking to feel sharper, less foggy, less like wading through something that was not there a decade ago.

These are not separate problems. They share a common cause: bodies that have stopped receiving the deliberate, varied, attentive movement they need. And they respond to a common solution, which is exactly what this program provides.

The 28-day plan in Chapter Five is structured in four weeks, each with a clear purpose. The early weeks ask very little. The later weeks ask more. There are two rest days each week, placed at the right points in the schedule to let the body consolidate what the practice days have built. Chapter Six explains what happens during those rest days in simple terms, because understanding it will change how you think about them.

Each practice session in this program runs for ten to twelve minutes. Not because I think that is all you are capable of. Because a daily twelve-minute habit that you maintain across four weeks produces more genuine change than a forty-minute session you do twice and abandon. Short, consistent, and attentive beats long, occasional, and distracted every time.

You will need a firm chair with a stable base, enough room around it to move your arms freely, and comfortable clothing that does not restrict your shoulders. You will not need anything else.

Read Chapter Three before you begin Day 1 of the program. It has three short tests that take about five minutes to complete. They establish your starting point for balance, joint stiffness, and focused attention. Without those starting numbers, the progress checks in Chapter Five cannot tell you how far you have come.

The chair is not a lesser version of the exercise mat. It is a platform with specific advantages for the work that needs doing in a body that has been through sixty or more years of life. My grandmother understood that. She practiced every morning until she could not. This program is for the people who are still going.

Liuhe Chen

Before You Begin

A few practical matters to sort out before Day 1. Each one is short. All of them will make the program easier to follow.

Checking In With Your Doctor

Have a brief conversation with your doctor before you start if any of the following are true for you: you had surgery in the last six months; you have a heart condition that requires supervised exercise; a doctor has recommended against putting load through your shoulders, elbows, or hips; you have advanced bone thinning of the spine or upper limbs; you have a condition that affects your coordination or your ability to sit upright for a sustained period.

These exercises are gentle and chair-based. For most people over 60, there is no barrier to starting. But your doctor has context about your body that this book does not have, and a short check-in takes less time than any session in this program.

A distinction worth making early: mild joint warmth and a sense of muscle effort during the exercises are normal and expected. They are signs that the movement is reaching the joints and muscles it is designed to reach. Sharp pain, particularly pain that is localized to a specific joint, is a different signal. If you feel sharp pain during any exercise, stop. Rest. Do not continue that exercise until you have spoken to a doctor.

Setting Up Your Chair

The chair matters more than most people think. Use a dining chair or kitchen chair with a firm, flat seat and a stable base. Not a rocking chair, not an office chair on wheels, not a low armchair where the seat cushion is soft enough to let the pelvis sink. The seat should be firm enough that you can feel the bones of your sitting position clearly.

Height is important. When you sit, your feet should rest flat on the floor with your knees roughly level with your hips. If the chair is slightly too high, place a folded blanket under your feet. If the chair is slightly too low, a firm cushion on the seat will raise your sitting position without making it unstable. Do not use a thick, soft cushion that compresses under your weight.

Arm rests are optional. Several exercises in Chapter Four are easier without them because they involve reaching to the side. If your chair has arm rests, you can still do those exercises, but your range may be slightly limited. If you have a choice of chairs, the one without arm rests is better for this program.

Place the chair with roughly two feet of clear space on each side so your arms can move freely. The floor under and around the chair should not be slippery. If you are on a smooth floor and the chair shifts, place a non-slip mat underneath it.

What to Wear

Wear clothes that allow your shoulders and arms to move through their full range. Stiff sleeves, a close-fitting jacket, or thick layering across the shoulders will limit the shoulder exercises. Flat-soled shoes or bare feet work better than thick-soled running shoes, which raise your center of gravity slightly and reduce the ground-feel that the foot and ankle exercises use.

How to Work Through This Book

Chapter One covers what seated practice can actually do for your body and why. Chapter Two explains the mechanisms behind the three benefits in plain terms. Chapter Three prepares your body for Day 1 and has the three baseline tests. Complete those before starting the 28-day program. The progress checks in Chapter Five compare directly to those starting numbers, so without them, the checks have no reference point.

Chapter Four contains all ten exercises written out fully with step-by-step instructions and illustrations. Spend a few minutes with each exercise before it shows up in the Chapter Five program. You do not need to commit them to memory. Seeing them once means that when Chapter Five directs you to a specific exercise by name, you arrive with a mental picture of it rather than starting from scratch.

Chapter Five is the daily program. Each practice day has a brief session summary, a coaching note from me, and a specific focus cue. Read the coaching note before the session, not after. It is short and it changes what you notice during the session.

Rest Days

Two rest days are built into each week of the 28-day program, eight rest days in total. They fall at specific points in the schedule, chosen for where the body benefits most from consolidation. The positions shift each week so that no single day becomes a habitual skip.

A rest day is not a day off from the program. It is a scheduled part of it. What the exercise days build, the rest days allow to settle. Chapter Six explains this in more detail. For now: honor the rest days. Do not replace them with a makeup session. Do not compress two days into one when a rest day falls inconveniently. The schedule is designed around the biology.

On rest days, light activity is fine. A slow walk, some gentle stretching, ordinary household movement. What a rest day is not: a formal practice session.

Pace

Every exercise in this program is slower than feels natural. This is the design, not a limitation. The joint benefit, the balance training, and the mental engagement that produce the three subtitle improvements all depend on deliberate slowness. Momentum is not your friend here. Attention is. When an exercise starts to feel comfortable at its current pace, the instruction is not to speed it up. The instruction is to pay closer attention to the quality of what is happening in your shoulder, or your breath, or your trunk, within the pace the exercise already uses.

The slowness will feel strange in Week One. By Week Two it will feel purposeful. By Week Three it will feel like your own.

Chapter 1

What Your Chair Can Do for You

There is a version of this conversation where I spend the first chapter apologizing for the chair. Explaining its limitations. Reassuring you that even though the exercises are seated, they are still worth doing. I am not going to do that. The chair is not a compromise. It is the right tool for a specific job, and this chapter explains why.

Why Seated Practice Is a Real Workout, Not a Shortcut

Most exercise instructions for seniors begin with a standing person and work backward from there. A standard balance exercise might ask you to stand on one leg. A standard strength exercise might ask you to stand and do a calf raise. When someone raises the concern that they cannot do those things safely, the response is usually a chair modification, something like: you can hold the back of the chair if you need to, or you can sit down and do a gentler version.

That approach starts in the wrong place. It starts with an exercise designed for one set of physical conditions and patches it for another. The result is a modified version of something, not something built with the right starting conditions in mind. When an exercise is built from the chair up, the design logic changes entirely. Instead of asking what can we reduce to make this safer, the question becomes what does this position make possible that standing does not.

Here is what a stable seated position makes possible. It removes the background work of standing balance. When you are upright and standing, a portion of your nervous system's attention is continuously occupied with keeping you from falling. That portion is not large, but it is not nothing. For a person whose standing balance is uncertain, or whose legs are under joint stress, or who is rebuilding confidence after a fall or an illness, that background work is significant. Removing it by sitting down does not remove the exercise. It relocates the exercise's full demand to the part of the body you are actually training.

For the shoulder exercises in this program, that matters enormously. The Arm Float, the Shoulder Roll and Open, the Side Reach, and the Chest Open and Close are all movements that ask the shoulder joint to work through a deliberate range with sustained attention. When you do those exercises from a chair, the shoulders get the full attention the session has to give. When you do equivalent movements while also managing standing balance, some of that attention is elsewhere. The chair produces a higher quality of specific training for the upper body than standing exercises of the same type, not a lower quality.

The same logic applies to the thoracic spine exercises in this program. Seated Twist and the mid-back movements work on the thoracic vertebral joints that rarely get deliberate attention in standing exercise programs. From a chair, with the lower body stable and supported, the trunk can rotate through a full and controlled arc without the lower back compensating for what the thoracic spine cannot do. The exercise reaches the joint it is designed to reach.

Seated practice is not a shortcut. It is a specific, purposeful choice about where to position the body to get the most from a particular kind of training. The exercises in this program were not adapted from standing positions. They were built for the chair.

The Three Problems This Program Solves

The subtitle names three things: better balance, stronger joints, and a sharper mind. Behind each of those phrases is a real, specific, common problem that most people over 60 will recognize from their own experience.

The balance problem is usually noticed for the first time in a small, specific moment. Reaching for something on a high shelf and realizing the reach felt less certain than it used to. Stepping off a curb and feeling a flicker of hesitation before committing the weight. Sitting on an uneven surface, a bus seat, a folding chair, and noticing that recovering from a small unexpected tilt required more effort than it should have. These moments tend to accumulate quietly before anyone names them as a pattern.

What they have in common is a change in proprioception. Proprioception is the body's internal sense of its own position. It is not sight or hearing. It is the sense that tells you where your arm is when your eyes are closed, that tells your body how much correction to apply when you start to drift in any direction. Proprioception lives in the small sensory receptors inside joints, tendons, and muscles. After sixty, those receptors tend to become less responsive, particularly in joints that are not being moved deliberately and regularly. The result is a nervous system working from a less precise map of the body's position, which produces the small uncertainties that accumulate into the pattern of wariness that many older adults recognize in themselves.

The seated exercises in this program address proprioception through the joints that seated balance most depends on: the shoulders, the trunk, and the upper spine. The Seated Weight Shift exercise is specifically designed to train the trunk receptors. The Arm Float works the shoulder joint receptors through a slow, controlled arc. These are not lower-body proprioception exercises, because this is not a lower-body program. It is a seated upper-body program, and it trains the proprioceptive system that seated balance requires.

The joint problem tends to arrive more loudly than the balance problem. Morning stiffness that takes longer to ease than it used to. Shoulder pain that appears when reaching overhead. A hip that aches after sitting for an hour in a car. A mid-back that protests when turning to look behind you. These complaints share a mechanism. Joints need regular, varied movement to stay lubricated. The cartilage lining the joint surfaces has no direct blood supply. It receives its nutrients through a physical process: being gently compressed and released as the joint moves. A joint that is not moved regularly enough, or not moved through enough of its available range, becomes a joint that is nutritionally undersupplied and inflammation-prone.

The slow deliberate exercises in this program move the most commonly problematic joints through ranges that ordinary daily activity does not reliably reach. The Shoulder Roll and Open addresses the rotational arc of the shoulder. The Seated Twist reaches the thoracic facet joints that rounded posture and prolonged sitting compress. The Knee Lift and Lower works the hip joint through a flexion arc that sitting with bent knees all day does not provide. These are not random choices. The exercise list was built around the specific joints that respond most consistently to gentle, regular, deliberate movement in this age group.

The balance problem deserves one more observation that most exercise programs miss entirely. The standard description of balance problems focuses on standing: not falling when walking, managing an uneven surface, navigating a step without hesitation. These are real and important goals. But there is a second kind of balance problem that receives almost no dedicated attention: seated balance. The ability to remain stable when reaching across a table, to stay settled when a vehicle seat shifts, to move the arm or trunk freely without needing the other hand to anchor. Seated balance problems are as common and as limiting as standing balance problems in this age group. This program is built specifically to address them.

The mind problem is the one that people are most reluctant to name directly. Foggy thinking. Words that take longer to arrive. Difficulty holding a thought while dealing with a distraction. A sense that processing things is slower than it used to be. These experiences are common, real, and often attributed simply to age, as if they were as inevitable as gray hair.

Some of what older adults experience as cognitive slowing is driven by elevated cortisol. Cortisol is the body's primary stress hormone. When it is chronically elevated, which it often is in people managing pain, reduced mobility, and the anxiety that goes with both, it interferes with the part of the brain responsible for clear thinking, working memory, and focused attention. The slow, breath-coordinated movement of the exercises in this program is one of the most reliable ways to lower cortisol through non-pharmaceutical means. It activates the calm branch of the nervous system. Over weeks of daily practice, it shifts the hormonal baseline in a direction that produces measurable improvements in cognitive clarity. This is not a side effect. It is a primary mechanism.

How 10 Minutes a Day Creates Lasting Change

The number that surprises most people when they hear it is not the number of exercises. It is the session length. Ten to twelve minutes. That, people assume, cannot be enough.

The assumption behind that reaction is that exercise works by accumulating time. The longer the session, the more the body changes. This is true for some goals, most notably cardiovascular fitness. But for the three things this program addresses, balance, joint mobility, and cognitive clarity, the mechanism is different. These outcomes are produced by specificity and frequency, not by duration.

Proprioceptive training works by giving the joint receptors repeated, precise stimulation. A twelve-minute session of deliberate arm and trunk movement gives the shoulder, elbow, and spinal receptors that stimulation daily. A thirty-minute session done three times a week gives the same receptors less total daily contact time. For the nervous system, which learns through repetition and consolidates during rest, daily shorter sessions outperform infrequent longer ones.

Joint lubrication works by moving fluid through cartilage. A slow ten-minute session of varied joint movement is enough to produce the fluid circulation the cartilage needs. Extending the session to thirty minutes does not triple the benefit. The cartilage reaches its nutritional update within the first portion of the movement and does not receive proportionally more from additional time. What produces better joint outcomes is daily movement, not longer movement.

The cortisol reduction that produces mental clarity occurs within the first few minutes of slow breath-coordinated movement. The reduction is meaningful and measurable within a ten-minute session. The compounding effect of daily cortisol reduction, building over weeks, is what shifts the baseline and produces the sustained clarity improvement. One long session does not produce the same baseline shift as twenty daily shorter ones.

There is one more thing that shorter daily sessions produce that longer infrequent ones do not: a lower day-to-day variation in what the body receives. Biological systems that receive consistent moderate daily stimulation adapt more smoothly than those receiving large periodic doses. Joints moved gently every day build synovial health more reliably than joints exercised heavily twice a week and ignored otherwise. Proprioceptive receptors trained daily consolidate their learning more efficiently than those trained in weekend bursts. Consistency is not just a motivational virtue in this program. It is a physiological requirement for the outcomes the program is designed to produce.

The duration was also chosen for a reason that has nothing to do with physiology: twelve minutes is reliably achievable every day. It does not require a special window of time. It does not require a level of energy that some days do not have. It does not require a motivation level that varies with mood and circumstance. It requires a chair, twelve minutes, and the decision to start. That is the full ask. Programs that make a smaller daily ask produce more consistent behavior than those that make a larger occasional one. Consistency, across this program, is the variable that matters most.

Who This Book Is For

This program is written for adults over 60 who want to move better, hurt less, and think more clearly but need or prefer to do that work from a chair. It is for people who have reduced their daily movement because of joint pain, because of a fall or a long illness, because standing exercise programs have felt too demanding or too risky to sustain. It is for people using a wheelchair or a walker who want a structured daily practice that works within those conditions. It is for people who have been meaning to start something and have not found a starting point that actually fits.

It is also for people in perfectly good physical condition who want the specific benefits of slow, deliberate, chair-based practice. Some of the most consistent practitioners of this kind of work are people who could manage a standing program with no difficulty. They choose the chair because of what the chair offers: precision, safety margin, and the quality of attention that comes from removing the standing balance demand from the equation. That is a legitimate choice, not a sign of limitation.

A note for adult children or caregivers choosing this book for an older family member: the exercises are designed to be followed independently by the person who will be doing them. They do not require supervision. They do not require a trained instructor. The instructions and illustrations are clear enough for a person sitting alone in their kitchen chair on a Tuesday morning to follow without guidance. If the practitioner wants company or coaching during the sessions, that is welcome. If they prefer to practice alone, the book supports that equally well.

This book does not require any background in Tai Chi. It does not require any particular level of fitness or any prior experience with structured exercise. The exercises are described in plain language with clear illustrations. The instructions are meant to be followed by someone sitting in their kitchen chair on a Tuesday morning who has not exercised in years. If the exercises are readable and the chair is stable, the program is accessible.

It is worth being clear about something that often goes unsaid in books like this. The exercises are simple. They are meant to be simple. They are not simple because this program thinks you are incapable of complexity. They are simple because simplicity is a design choice that produces better results for the goals this program has. A complex exercise that is hard to remember and awkward to perform is a worse proprioceptive training tool than a simple exercise done with full attention and consistent form. The value is in the quality of the repetition, not in the impressiveness of the movement. Simple exercises done well, every day, for four weeks, produce genuine changes. That is the design.

One thing to know before you start: this program is honest about what it will and will not do. It will improve the specific things it trains: seated balance, joint mobility in the targeted areas, and cognitive clarity through cortisol reduction and attention training. It will not rebuild seriously damaged cartilage, restore neurological conditions that affect motor function, or produce cardiovascular fitness gains of the kind running or cycling provide. Those boundaries are not failures. They are the correct scope of a program designed around a specific population and three specific outcomes. Knowing the scope helps you recognize the progress when it arrives, which it will.

Chapter 2

How Seated Tai Chi Works

The exercises in this program produce three specific benefits. Each benefit comes from a specific mechanism. This chapter explains each one in ordinary language so that when you feel the effects of the practice, you understand what is causing them and why continuing the practice is the right response to those effects.

The Science of Slow Movement and Joint Health

Every joint in your body is surrounded by a sealed capsule filled with fluid. That fluid is called synovial fluid, and it does two jobs that nothing else in the joint can do. It lubricates the surfaces where two bones meet so that the cartilage can slide against itself without grinding. And it feeds the cartilage, which has no blood vessels of its own and cannot receive nutrients any other way.

The way synovial fluid feeds cartilage is through pressure. When the joint is gently loaded and then released, the cartilage compresses slightly, squeezing out used fluid, and then expands, drawing in fresh fluid loaded with the nutrients the cartilage cells need to stay healthy. This exchange only happens when the joint moves. A joint held still for hours, which is what most older adults do for much of their day, receives very little of this exchange. The cartilage becomes nutritionally starved. Waste products accumulate. The joint stiffens, becomes inflamed, and hurts more than it would if it had been moving regularly.

This is why so many people with joint pain feel worst after rest. The overnight stillness of sleep, the hours of sitting in a chair, the lack of varied movement through the joint's full range, all reduce the fluid exchange the cartilage depends on. The stiffness and aching of the first twenty minutes of a morning are the joints reporting that the exchange did not happen during the night.

Slow movement is the key ingredient for restoring this exchange. Fast movement carries the joint through its range too quickly for the fluid to distribute well. Slow movement, particularly movement that pauses at different points through the arc, gives the cartilage time to compress and expand fully at each position. This is why the exercises in this program are performed slowly, not just as a safety measure for people with balance concerns, but because the therapeutic benefit to the joint is highest at slow speeds. Moving faster would reduce the treatment, not intensify it.

The joints most commonly affected in this age group, the shoulders, thoracic spine, hips, and knees, are not equally addressed by all exercise programs. Programs focused on walking reach the lower joints but leave the shoulder and upper back largely untouched. Programs designed purely for the upper body often omit the hip and knee work that seated movement can provide through exercises like the Knee Lift and Lower and the Heel Raise Seated. The exercises in this program are mapped specifically to cover all of these areas within each session.

A second mechanism that affects joints is inflammation. Joints that are inflamed hurt more, move less, and stiffen faster. The main driver of chronic low-level joint inflammation in older adults is not always structural damage inside the joint. A significant portion of it is driven by chronically elevated cortisol, the body's stress hormone. Cortisol promotes pro-inflammatory signalling throughout the body. When cortisol is high for extended periods, joints that might otherwise manage their inflammation reasonably well become significantly more symptomatic. The breath-coordinated movement of the exercises in this program lowers cortisol measurably within a session and shifts the baseline lower over weeks of daily practice. The joint that was hurting partly because of cortisol-driven inflammation will hurt less not only because it is moving more but because the inflammatory environment it is sitting in has improved.

Balance From the Chair Up

Balance is commonly discussed as if it were entirely about the feet and legs. This is understandable, because the most dramatic consequences of poor balance, falls, are lower-body events. But the system that manages balance involves three separate inputs and the brain regions that integrate them. One of those inputs comes from the inner ear, which registers the head's position and movement. One comes from the eyes. And one comes from the proprioceptive sensors inside joints, muscles, and tendons throughout the entire body, not just the lower limbs.

For a person sitting in a chair, the proprioceptive inputs from the lower body are largely bypassed because the chair is managing the standing demand. What remains active are the proprioceptive inputs from the trunk, the shoulders, the upper spine, and the arms. These are the inputs that manage seated balance, the ability to reach without tipping, to turn without losing your position, to absorb the movement of a vehicle seat or a bus without grabbing for support.

The shoulder joint has a particularly dense network of proprioceptive receptors in its capsule and surrounding ligaments. When the shoulder moves slowly and deliberately through a range, those receptors send detailed position and movement information to the brain. This information contributes directly to the brain's real-time map of where the upper body is in space. A shoulder joint that is moved regularly and precisely gives the brain better information. A shoulder joint that is rarely moved through its full range gives the brain less information, and the seated balance that depends on upper body positioning becomes less reliable.

The Arm Float exercise, the Seated Weight Shift, and the Side Reach in this program are designed primarily around this mechanism. They are not just stretching exercises. They are proprioceptive training sessions for the shoulder, trunk, and thoracic spine receptors that manage seated stability. Each slow repetition of each exercise sends a fresh stream of position data to the brain. Over weeks of daily practice, the quality and reliability of that data stream improves. The seated balance that results is not a vague general improvement. It is the specific, measurable result of training specific sensors to do their job more accurately.

There is a transfer benefit to standing and walking that most people do not expect from chair-based practice. The trunk muscles and shoulder girdle muscles that maintain stable seated posture are the same muscles that maintain stable upright posture during standing and walking. Practitioners of this program consistently report improvements in how they feel on their feet as a secondary benefit of the seated training, because the trunk work is not position-specific. It transfers out of the chair.

How Breath and Gentle Motion Clear Mental Fog

The mental fog that many people over 60 describe is not one thing. Several different causes can produce similar-feeling cognitive symptoms. But one of the most consistent and most directly addressable contributors is elevated cortisol.

The brain region most responsible for what we experience as clear thinking, working memory, focused attention, and quick word retrieval is the prefrontal cortex. It is also the region most densely packed with cortisol receptors. When cortisol is elevated, the prefrontal cortex receives a sustained chemical signal that reduces its efficiency. Thoughts feel harder to hold. Attention drifts more easily. Words take longer to surface. Tasks that used to feel effortless require more mental energy than they should. This is not a structural decline in the brain. It is a functional response to a hormonal environment. Change the environment, and the function improves.

The slow breathing pattern that accompanies every exercise in this program is one of the most reliable ways to change that environment quickly. When you breathe in slowly through the nose and exhale slowly through slightly parted lips, you stimulate the vagus nerve, which is the main cable of the parasympathetic nervous system. The parasympathetic system is the calm, repair branch of the autonomic nervous system. Its activation suppresses cortisol production, slows the heart rate slightly, relaxes the muscular tension that chronic stress accumulates, and shifts the prefrontal cortex out of its high-cortisol, low-performance state. Most people notice a recognizable mental shift within the first few minutes of a session. That shift is real and it is physiological.

The cognitive engagement of the exercises adds a second mechanism. Following a sequence of slow deliberate movements requires the working memory to hold the next step while executing the current one. It requires the attention to stay with what the body is doing rather than drifting to whatever else is competing for mental space. It requires the spatial awareness to track where the arms are moving and what happens next. These are genuine executive function demands. They are the same kinds of demands that mental puzzles and memory games use, but they are delivered through the body, which adds the proprioceptive and physiological benefits that sitting at a table with a pencil and paper cannot.

After several weeks of daily practice, most people notice a quality of thinking outside the sessions that was simply not there before. Faster word retrieval. Easier concentration through conversations or tasks that previously required more effort. A calmer quality to the day. These are not imagined improvements. They are the downstream effects of daily cortisol reduction compounding into a lower hormonal baseline, better sleep quality, and a prefrontal cortex that is doing its job in a friendlier chemical environment than it was operating in before.

What Changes Week by Week

The three benefits do not all arrive on the same day. They develop on slightly different timelines, and knowing roughly what to expect when helps you recognize progress rather than dismissing it because it does not look like what you were watching for.

The first week is mostly about learning. Your brain is building the motor programs for the ten exercises. This is actual cognitive work, the same kind of learning load that any new skill creates. Sessions may feel more mentally demanding than physically demanding. The movements may feel awkward. Your breath may keep falling out of coordination with the exercises. None of this is a problem. It is exactly what Week One is supposed to produce. The learning load decreases as the week progresses.

In Week Two, the joint effects begin to arrive. The daily fluid movement through the shoulder and thoracic joints accumulates into a noticeable change in morning stiffness. Most people who practice consistently through Week Two report that the first twenty minutes of their day start to feel different. The joints that were loudest in the morning quiet down faster. The shoulders that required fifteen minutes of careful movement before the day felt possible start to feel more ready within ten. This is the synovial fluid mechanism working.

Week Three brings the balance and clarity improvements into sharper focus. The proprioceptive training has now had two weeks to accumulate. The brain's map of the upper body's position has become more detailed. People notice reaching further without bracing, turning more freely in their chair, feeling more settled in vehicle seats and on uneven surfaces. The cognitive changes that began building in Week Two become more consistently available across the full day rather than appearing only during or immediately after sessions.

Week Four is where the three changes begin to feel like one thing rather than three separate developments. Clearer thinking makes it easier to sustain attention through the exercises. Better attention during the exercises deepens the proprioceptive training and the joint benefit. Reduced joint stiffness means the exercises can be done with fuller range, which deepens both the fluid circulation and the proprioceptive signal. The system that produces the three benefits has been running for three weeks. In Week Four it begins to feel like a system rather than like three separate efforts.

Day 28 marks the end of the program and the beginning of a practice that now has a history behind it. What has been built in four weeks does not disappear if the program stops. It persists and continues to develop as long as the daily sessions continue. The progress check on Day 28 is not a final score. It is a measurement of a practice that is still in motion.

<h1 style="text-align:center">Chapter 3</h1>

<h1 style="text-align:center">Before You Sit Down to Practice</h1>

The few minutes you spend on this chapter before Day 1 will pay back every session that follows. Get the chair right. Do the baseline tests. Understand what the body scan is for. Then you will be ready to start.

Picking the Right Chair

The chair is your equipment. The quality of your practice depends on getting it right.

The seat must be firm and flat. When you sit, you need to feel the bones of your pelvis making clear contact with the seat. If the seat is soft or cushioned enough that you sink into it, your pelvis tilts backward, your lower back rounds, and the trunk control that the exercises depend on becomes significantly harder to access. A wooden dining chair or a firm kitchen chair with minimal cushioning is ideal. If all your chairs have soft seats, place a firm, non-compressible cushion on top of the softest one before using it for practice.

The seat height matters. When seated with your feet flat on the floor, your knees should be at roughly the same height as your hips, creating approximately a right angle at the knee. If the chair is too high and your feet dangle, place a folded blanket or a firm, flat footrest under your feet before starting any session. If the chair is too low and your knees sit higher than your hips, a firm non-slip seat cushion will bring the sitting height up. Both adjustments take less than a minute and make a meaningful difference to how the exercises feel and work.

Arm rests are not ideal for this program. Most of the exercises involve reaching the arms out to the sides or forward without obstruction. If your best available chair has fixed arm rests, you can still use it, but you will find that the Side Reach and the Arm Float exercises have reduced range. If you have a choice, use the chair without arm rests for practice sessions.

Setting Up Your Space

The space directly around the chair also needs to be clear. Extend both arms fully to the sides and then forward. Nothing should obstruct that range of motion. A clear radius of about two feet on each side is sufficient. The floor directly under the chair should not be slippery. If you are on a smooth floor, place a rubber-backed mat under the chair legs to keep it from sliding during exercises that involve a strong lean or reach.

Natural light is a nice addition but not required. Consistent session timing helps the habit embed, so wherever the chair is positioned, it should be somewhere you can get to easily at the same time each day. A space you have to rearrange furniture to access will create friction that a space you walk straight into will not.

5-Minute Body Scan Before Any Session

Begin every practice session with this brief check, not just in Week One, every session across all four weeks. It takes about two minutes and serves two purposes: it brings your attention into the body before the exercises begin, and it gives you the information you need to adapt the session if something is more symptomatic than usual.

Sit in your chair. Feet flat. Back away from the chair back so you are sitting on your own support rather than leaning. Take one slow breath in and one slow breath out before you start.

Neck and shoulders:

Turn your head slowly to the right as far as it goes comfortably, then back to center, then to the left. Note whether one side is tighter or more restricted than the other. Roll both shoulders up toward your ears, then back and down, making a slow backward circle. Do this twice. Note whether either shoulder has more resistance than usual, any clicking, or any uncomfortable catching sensation.

Arms and elbows:

Extend both arms forward at shoulder height, palms facing each other. Hold for three seconds. Lower. Note whether either arm feels noticeably heavier, weaker, or more resistant than the other. Bend both elbows and bring your hands toward your shoulders. Note any restriction or discomfort at the elbow joint.

Lower back and hips:

Place both hands on your thighs. Sit tall and then gently lean forward from the hips until you feel a mild stretch in the lower back. Return to upright. Note any significant tightness, pulling, or discomfort. Then gently place both hands on the outside of one knee and pull it slightly toward your chest. Hold two seconds. Repeat on the other side. Note any hip restriction or groin discomfort.

Feet and ankles:

Lift both heels slowly, pressing the toes into the floor. Lower. Then lift both toes, pressing the heels into the floor. Do each three times. Note any ankle stiffness, swelling, or unusual discomfort in the feet.

After the scan, you have a current picture of how the body is presenting today. If something is notably more symptomatic than usual, you can reduce the range of the exercises that use that area, or substitute the Easier Option for those exercises that day. This is not avoidance. It is informed practice.

The body scan also trains something less tangible: the habit of turning attention inward before movement begins. One of the distinguishing features of this kind of practice is that it asks you to pay attention to what the body is reporting rather than simply executing a movement regardless of what the body is doing. That attentiveness is a skill. The body scan is the five-minute daily practice of it. By Week Three, many people find that the scan has made them generally more perceptive about their own physical state throughout the day, not just in the session.

It is also worth noting what the body scan is not. It is not a full health assessment. It is not a reason to stop if everything is not feeling perfect. Some level of morning stiffness, mild joint resistance, and general low energy is the normal starting state for many older adults and is not a barrier to practicing. The scan is designed to identify significant changes from your baseline, not to screen for universal readiness. Minor discomfort is expected. Sharp pain is the signal that warrants a modification.

Seated Posture, Foot Position, and Breath Basics

Every exercise in this program begins from the same starting position. Learning it well before Day 1 means you will not be learning posture and exercises simultaneously on Day 1.

Sitting position:

Sit at the front half of the chair seat, not leaning back against the chair back. Your sitting bones, the two bony points at the base of your pelvis, should be making clear contact with the seat. Feet flat on the floor, hip-width apart. Knees at roughly a right angle. Spine upright without being strained. Imagine a thread pulling the top of your head gently toward the ceiling. Shoulders relaxed away from the ears, not pulled back aggressively or hunched forward.

This posture will feel like mild effort at first, particularly in the mid-back and lower core. That is correct. Those muscles are being asked to do something they may not have been asked to do in a long time. By Week Two, the posture will require noticeably less active effort, and the muscles that felt strained holding it will have strengthened enough to make it feel natural.

If the upright posture produces lower back pain rather than mild muscular effort, check that you are not forcing the lumbar spine into an exaggerated arch. The instruction is a long, neutral spine, not a pressed-back posture. Think of sitting tall from the top of the head rather than from the base of the spine. If lower back pain persists during seated upright practice, use a rolled towel behind the lower back as a light support while the postural muscles build. Remove it for the final week of the program.

Foot position:

Both feet flat on the floor, hip-width apart, toes pointing roughly forward. The soles of the feet should make full contact with the floor, not just the ball of the foot or just the heel. The pressure should feel fairly even across the whole sole. Noticing foot pressure is the first form of seated balance awareness this program develops.

Breathing:

The breathing pattern used through all ten exercises is the same: slow in through the nose, slow out through the mouth. The exhale should be longer than the inhale. A useful rhythm is to inhale for a count of three and exhale for a count of four or five. The exhale does not need to be forceful. It should feel like a controlled, slow release rather than a push.

Before you start each session, take three full breaths in this pattern before beginning the first exercise. These three breaths are not optional. They are the transition from ordinary daily activity into the quality of attention the exercises need. Every session in Chapter Five begins with them.

Your Starting Point: Three Simple Baseline Tests

Complete these three tests before Day 1. Record the results. They are the reference numbers for the progress checks on Days 14, 21, and 28.

Test One: Seated Arm-Hold for Balance

1. Sit in your practice chair in the standard starting position.

2. Raise your right arm directly in front of you to shoulder height, palm facing down.

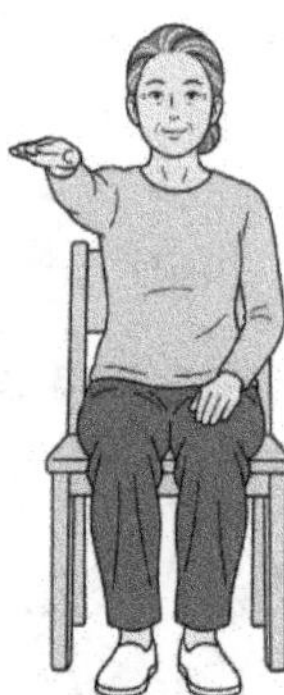

3. Hold the position without letting the arm drift down for as long as you can while keeping the arm level. Count the seconds silently.

4. Lower the arm when it begins to drop. Record the time for the right arm.

5. Rest for thirty seconds, then repeat with the left arm. Record the time.

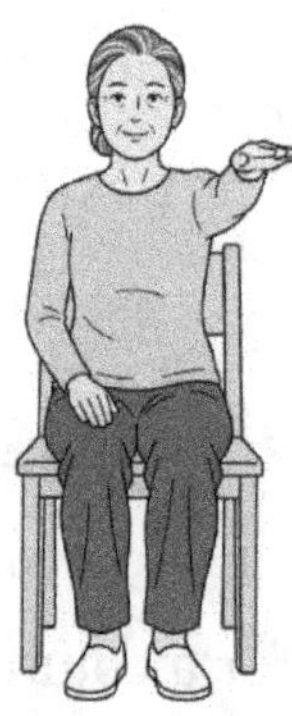

6. These times are your Day 1 seated arm-hold baseline for BALANCE.

Test Two: Morning Joint Stiffness Rating

On three consecutive mornings before Day 1, immediately after waking and before getting out of bed, rate how stiff your joints feel on a scale of one to five. One means no stiffness at all. Five means significant stiffness that limits how freely you can move until it eases. Focus particularly on your shoulders, hands, hips, and knees.

Average the three morning ratings. This average is your Day 1 joint stiffness baseline for JOINTS.

Test Three: Focused Attention Check

1. Sit quietly without music, television, or phone notifications.
2. Set a timer for three minutes.
3. Count backward from one hundred by sevens: one hundred, ninety-three, eighty-six, seventy-nine, and so on.
4. Every time your attention drifts away from the counting and you have to find your place again, make a small mark on a piece of paper.
5. When the timer ends, count the marks. That number is your Day 1 attention-drift score for MIND.
6. A lower score on Day 28 means the practice has improved your focused attention.

Keep these three numbers somewhere easy to find. The progress checks in Chapter Five refer back to them directly.

One important note about these tests: there are no right or wrong scores. These tests are not competitive and they are not a screen for whether you are well enough to do this program. They are a personal baseline. A short arm-hold time on Day 1 is not a failure. It is a starting point. A high attention-drift count on Day 1 is not a reflection of cognitive decline. It is where the practice begins. The value of the tests is entirely in the comparison between Day 1 and Day 28, not in the numbers themselves.

Chapter 4

The Chair Exercises

Ten exercises. Each one is described in full with step-by-step instructions and illustrations. Read through every exercise before Day 1 so that Chapter Five can refer to them by name and you already know roughly what each one looks like.

How to Follow the Instructions

Each exercise block is laid out the same way. The exercise name appears as a heading. Below it is a single line explaining which of the three subtitle benefits, balance, joints, or sharpened mind, this exercise primarily targets. Then the image prompts, followed by the numbered steps. Steps always restart at 1 for each new exercise.

After the steps, four cue lines give you the most important things to pay attention to: BREATHING, FEEL IT, JOINT BENEFIT, and BALANCE TIP. These are the one-line versions of what the exercise is for. Read them before doing the exercise the first time.

The EASIER OPTION at the end of each block describes a reduced-range version for days when full range is not accessible, whether because of pain, fatigue, or simply being early in the program before the range has built. The Easier Option delivers the same benefit at a smaller scale. It is not a lesser exercise. It is the correct exercise for those conditions.

The images show the character at the start position and at a key point mid-exercise. In some exercises, a third image shows the end position. The illustrations are line-art style, consistent in character appearance throughout the book. No text labels or callouts appear on the images. Where a movement direction is not obvious from the body position alone, a single solid black arrow indicates the direction. Arrows are used sparingly and only where the direction genuinely needs clarification.

A note on how to use the images and the steps together: read the numbered steps first, then look at the image for the corresponding position, then do the step. This read-see-do sequence builds the motor program more effectively than simply watching an image and trying to copy it. The steps give you the internal instructions. The images give you the external reference. Both together are more useful than either alone.

The Ten Chair Exercises

Exercise 1: Settle and Breathe

Primary benefit: SHARPER MIND. This exercise starts every session. It lowers cortisol, activates the calm branch of the nervous system, and shifts attention from daily thoughts into the body where it needs to be.

1. Sit in the starting position. Feet flat, hip-width apart. Hands resting on thighs. Back straight, shoulders down.

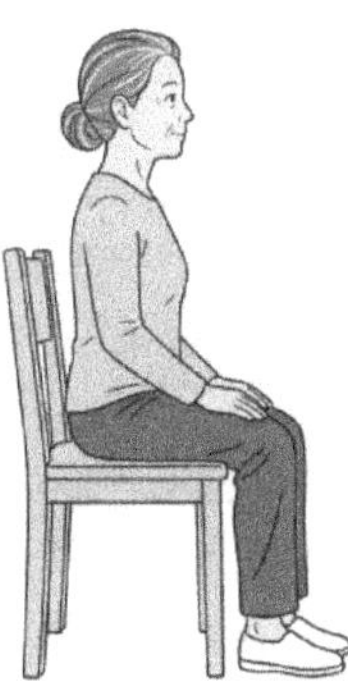

2. Close your eyes or soften your gaze toward the floor.
3. Breathe in slowly through your nose for a count of three. Feel the breath fill the belly first, then the chest.
4. Breathe out slowly through slightly parted lips for a count of five. Let the chest and belly soften.
5. Repeat this breath cycle four more times, five cycles in total.
6. After the fifth exhale, open your eyes. You are ready for the first exercise.

BREATHING: This exercise is only breathing. Each exhale is longer than the inhale. Do not rush the exhale.

FEEL IT: A mild heaviness in the hands and a slight softening across the chest and upper back as the breathing continues. This is the nervous system beginning to settle.

JOINT BENEFIT: The extended exhale reduces cortisol, which lowers background joint inflammation throughout the body.

BALANCE TIP: Notice how evenly your weight is distributed across both sitting bones right now. This awareness is the foundation of seated balance.

EASIER OPTION
If five full cycles feels like too many at first, start with three. The quality of each breath matters more than the number.

Exercise 2: Arm Float

Primary benefit: BETTER BALANCE. Trains the shoulder joint receptors that manage seated upper body stability, the proprioceptive system that keeps you from tipping when reaching or turning.

1. From the starting position, inhale slowly.

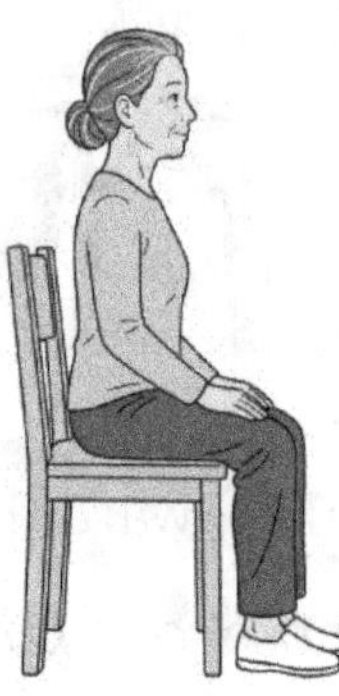

2. As you inhale, let both arms rise in front of you as if they are being lifted by the breath, palms facing down. Move slowly. The arms should reach shoulder height by the end of the inhale.

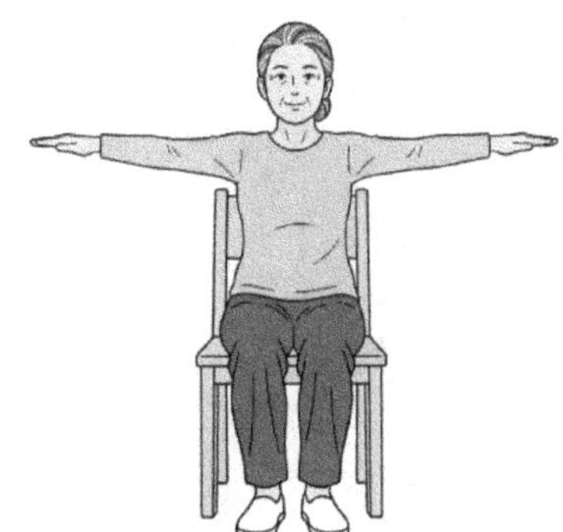

3. Hold at the top for two seconds. Keep breathing.

4. Exhale slowly. Let the arms lower back to the thighs at the same pace as the exhale.

5. Repeat six times.

BREATHING: Inhale as the arms rise. Exhale as they lower. The breath leads the movement, not the other way around.

FEEL IT: A mild awareness inside the shoulder joint as the arm rises. Not effort in the muscles, but a quality of the joint moving through its range. That awareness is proprioception activating.

JOINT BENEFIT: The slow arc through the shoulder range distributes synovial fluid through the superior joint space, the area most affected by rounded shoulders.

BALANCE TIP: As the arms rise, notice whether your trunk stays level or whether one side lifts slightly with the arms. Keeping the trunk still while the arms move is a seated balance skill.

> **EASIER OPTION**
> Raise only one arm at a time if both together is uncomfortable. Alternate right and left, six times each.

Exercise 3: Shoulder Roll and Open

Primary benefit: STRONGER JOINTS. Moves the shoulder joint through its rotational arc and opens the chest, reversing the closed, rounded posture that leads to shoulder stiffness and upper back tightness.

1. Lift both shoulders up toward your ears slowly.

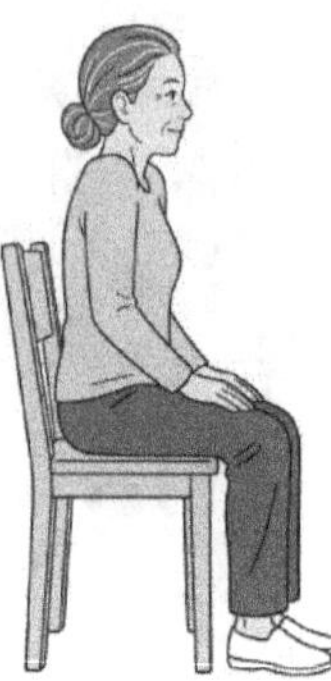

2. Roll them back, squeezing the shoulder blades gently together at the back.

3. Drop the shoulders down away from the ears.

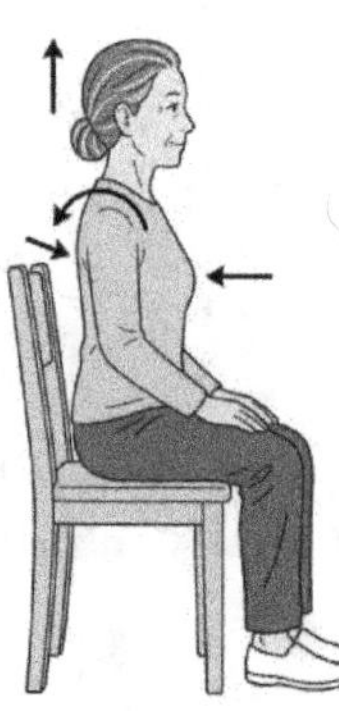

4. Roll them forward and then up again to complete the circle. This is one full backward roll.

5. Complete four backward rolls slowly.

6. Reverse direction: lift up, roll forward, drop down, roll back. Complete four forward rolls.

7. After the last roll, let the shoulders settle naturally in their lowest, most relaxed position.

BREATHING: Inhale as the shoulders rise. Exhale as they drop and roll through the lower part of the circle.

FEEL IT: A sense of motion inside the shoulder joints, particularly at the back and top of the arc. Any clicking or grinding that does not come with pain is the joint moving through a range it does not often use.

JOINT BENEFIT: The circular motion reaches the shoulder capsule in directions that most daily activity never does, distributing synovial fluid throughout the joint.

BALANCE TIP: Keep the trunk completely still during the shoulder rolls. Only the shoulders move. This stability is an active balance task.

EASIER OPTION
Make smaller circles if the full range produces discomfort. Smaller circles are still effective for joint lubrication.

Exercise 4: Seated Weight Shift

Primary benefit: BETTER BALANCE. Directly trains the trunk receptors that manage seated stability by moving the body's weight from one side to the other in a slow, controlled arc.

1. Place both hands on your thighs. Sit tall.

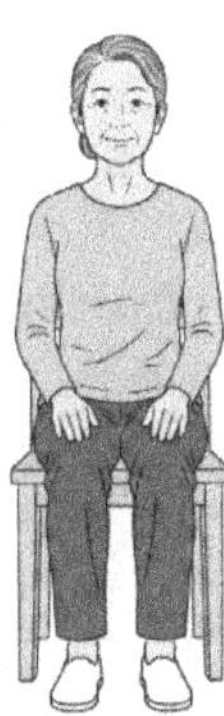

2. Slowly shift your weight to the right. Let the right hip drop slightly and the left hip lift slightly as the weight moves right. Your trunk tilts gently right.

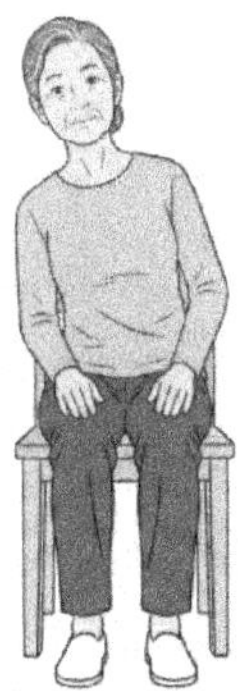

3. Hold the right position for two seconds. Feel the weight through the right sitting bone clearly.

4. Slowly return through center and continue shifting left. Hold left for two seconds.

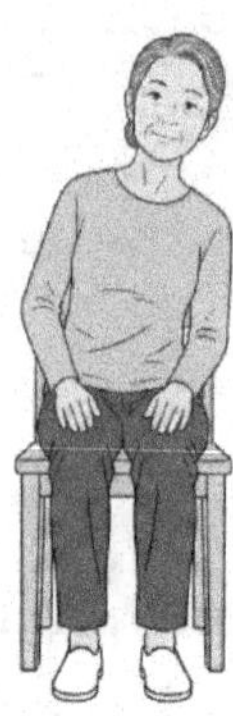

5. Return to center. This is one full cycle.

6. Complete six cycles, moving slowly and with full control in each direction.

BREATHING: Exhale as you shift to each side. Inhale as you return through center.

FEEL IT: The weight shifting clearly from one sitting bone to the other. In the first few sessions this shift may feel unsteady or unequal between sides. That unevenness is what the exercise is training.

JOINT BENEFIT: The lateral shift loads and unloads the hip joints on alternating sides, stimulating synovial fluid distribution through the hip capsule.

BALANCE TIP: Keep both feet flat on the floor throughout. Do not let the foot of the unweighted side lift as the weight shifts. Keeping both feet down is a stability anchor.

EASIER OPTION
Reduce the range of the shift until you find a degree of tilt that is controlled and comfortable. Even a small shift delivers the training benefit.

Exercise 5: Knee Lift and Lower

Primary benefit: STRONGER JOINTS. Works the hip flexors and lubricates the hip joint in the flexion arc that prolonged sitting suppresses, reducing the hip stiffness that many older adults feel when standing up from a chair.

1. Place both hands lightly on the tops of your thighs for light support.

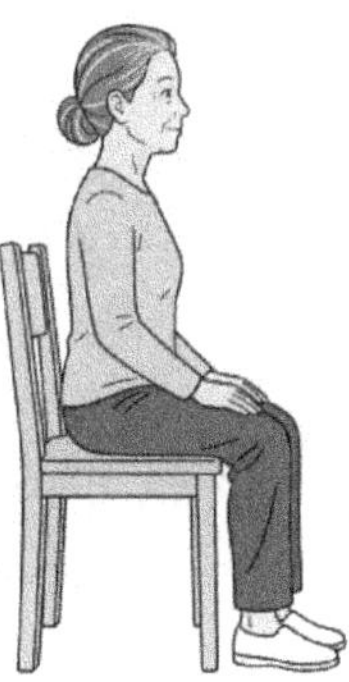

2. Slowly lift your right knee, raising the right foot a few inches from the floor.

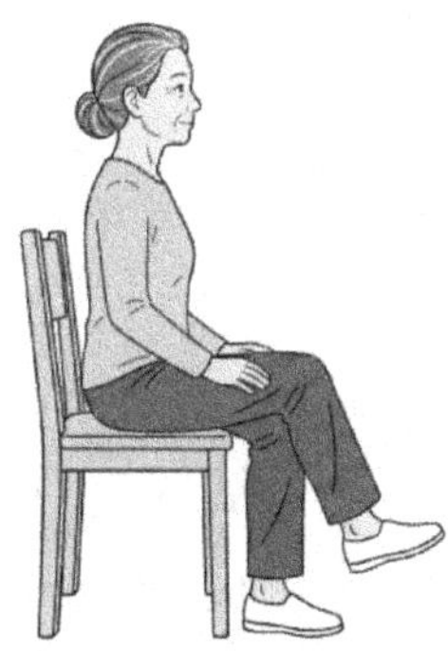

3. Hold the raised position for three seconds.

4. Lower the right foot slowly back to the floor with control.

5. Repeat on the left side: lift left knee

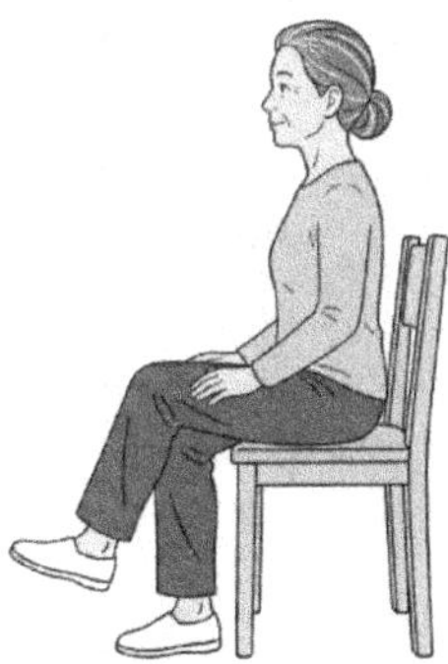

Hold three seconds and lower with control.

6. Alternate right and left for eight repetitions on each side.

BREATHING: Inhale as you lift the knee. Exhale during the hold. Inhale again as you lower.

FEEL IT: A mild effort in the front of the hip and upper thigh as the knee lifts. After several repetitions, a sense of warmth developing in the hip joint is the synovial fluid circulation beginning.

JOINT BENEFIT: Hip flexion loading provides the compression-release cycle the hip cartilage needs in a range that sitting with bent knees all day does not provide.

BALANCE TIP: Notice whether the trunk stays upright or whether it leans back as the knee rises. Keeping the trunk vertical while the hip flexes is a trunk control task.

> **EASIER OPTION**
> Reduce the height of the lift to just barely clearing the foot from the floor if full lift is uncomfortable. The hip flexion benefit is present at any lift height.

Exercise 6: Side Reach

Primary benefits: BETTER BALANCE and STRONGER JOINTS. Combines lateral trunk stability with a shoulder arc that lubricates the superior joint space while training the trunk receptors for sideways reach.

1. Sit tall. Place the left hand palm-down on the left thigh as a light anchor.

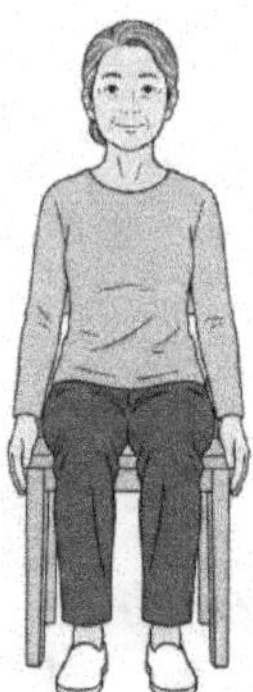

2. Slowly raise the right arm out to the right side in a wide arc, like a wing opening.

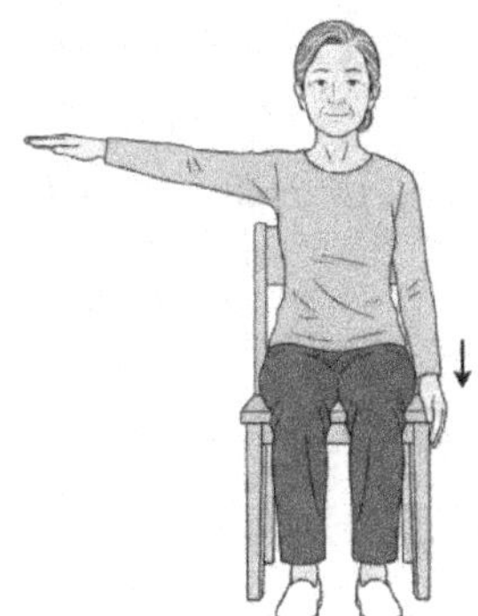

3. Continue raising the right arm overhead if comfortable, reaching toward the ceiling.

4. Hold at the top for two seconds.

5. Lower the right arm slowly back to the side, reversing the arc.

6. Repeat on the left side.

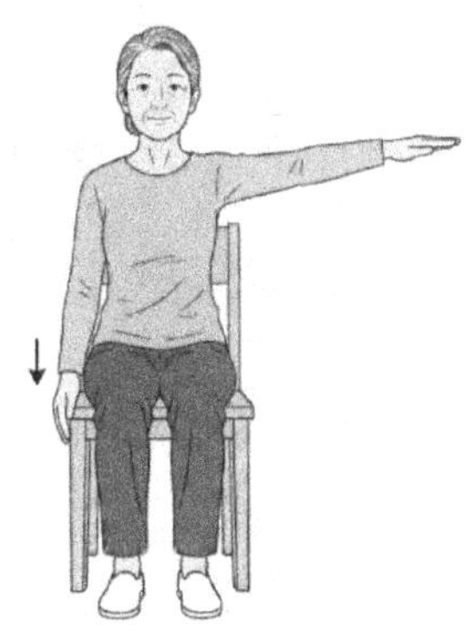

7. Alternate eight times on each side.

BREATHING: Inhale as the arm rises. Exhale as it lowers.

FEEL IT: A stretch along the side of the trunk as the arm reaches overhead, and a clear sense of the shoulder joint working through its upper arc.

JOINT BENEFIT: The overhead arc addresses the superior aspect of the shoulder joint and the upper thoracic spine, both areas where stiffness from forward posture accumulates.

BALANCE TIP: Keep the opposite hand anchored firmly on the thigh as a stability reference. The anchor hand is a deliberate balance cue, not just a resting hand.

EASIER OPTION

Raise the arm only to shoulder height rather than overhead if the full overhead reach is painful or restricted. The shoulder joint benefit is present at any height where the arm moves through a deliberate range.

Exercise 7: Chest Open and Close

Primary benefits: STRONGER JOINTS and SHARPER MIND. Opens the chest and thoracic spine while the paired breath pattern deepens the cortisol-reducing effect of the session.

1. Bring both hands to the center of the chest, elbows bent, fingertips touching lightly. This is the closed position.

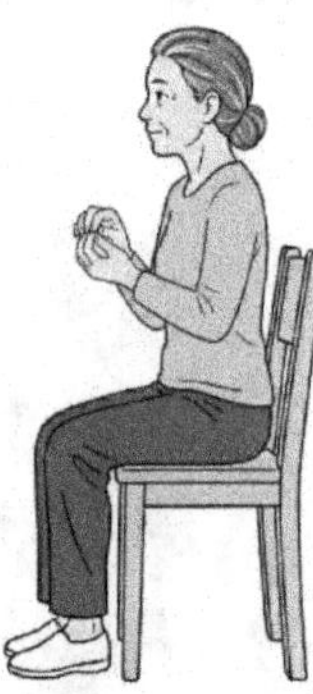

2. Inhale slowly. As you inhale, open the arms wide out to the sides, drawing the elbows back as if opening a book. Let the chest expand.

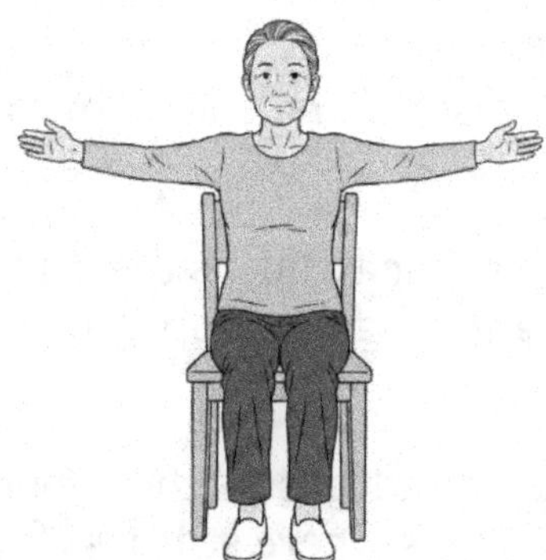

3. Hold the open position for one full exhale count, breathing out slowly.

4. Inhale and close: bring the elbows and fingertips back to center at the chest.

5. This is one full cycle. Complete eight cycles, moving slowly.

BREATHING: Inhale to open. Exhale to hold open. Inhale to close. Use the breath to drive the movement.

FEEL IT: A stretch through the pectorals and the front of the shoulders as the arms open. A sense of the upper back muscles engaging as the shoulder blades draw together.

JOINT BENEFIT: The opening arc mobilizes the thoracic facet joints and the anterior shoulder capsule, both areas compressed by prolonged forward-seated posture.

BALANCE TIP: Keep the trunk still and upright as the arms open. Do not let the opening pull the upper body backward or forward.

EASIER OPTION

Reduce the width of the open if full-range opening produces shoulder discomfort. Opening the arms to 45 degrees rather than full spread delivers the chest and thoracic benefit at reduced shoulder demand.

Exercise 8: Seated Twist

Primary benefits: STRONGER JOINTS and SHARPER MIND. Rotates the thoracic spine through a controlled arc that most daily activity never provides, reducing mid-back stiffness while requiring sustained focused attention to execute correctly.

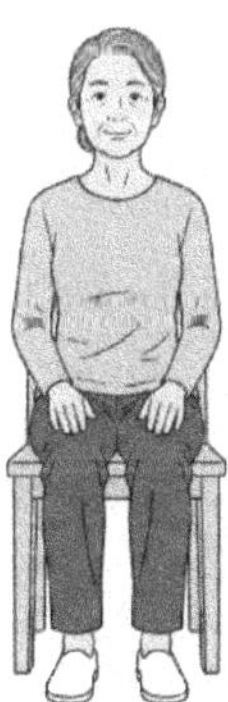

1. Cross your arms loosely over your chest, right hand on left shoulder, left hand on right shoulder.

2. Keeping the hips facing forward and both feet flat on the floor, slowly rotate your upper body to the right.

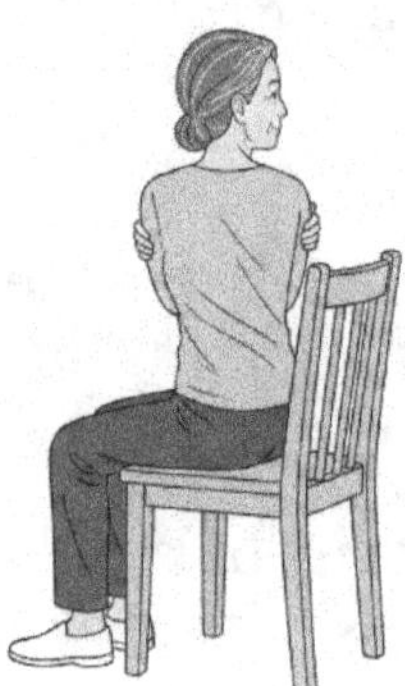

3. Rotate only as far as is comfortable without the hips twisting. Hold for three seconds.

4. Slowly return to the center.

5. Rotate to the left to the same degree. Hold three seconds.

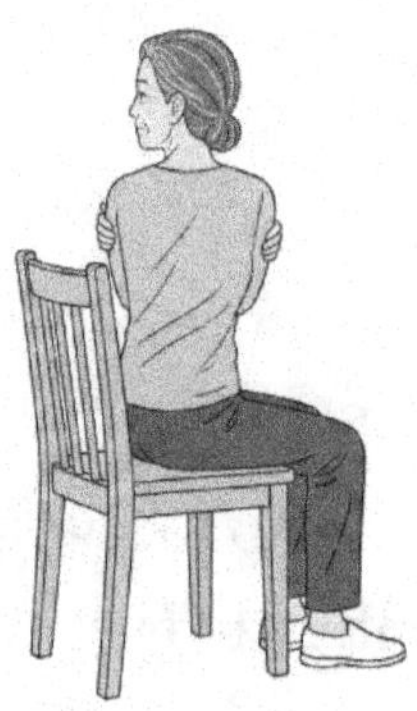

6. Return to center. This is one cycle. Complete six cycles.

BREATHING: Exhale as you rotate into the twist. Inhale as you return to center.

FEEL IT: A gentle wringing sensation through the mid-back as the thoracic spine rotates. The hips should feel anchored and still.

JOINT BENEFIT: Rotation is the movement the thoracic facet joints need most and receive least. This exercise directly addresses thoracic joint stiffness from prolonged forward-seated posture.

BALANCE TIP: The requirement to rotate the upper body while the lower body stays still is a trunk stability challenge. This is deliberate.

EASIER OPTION

Reduce the rotation range if the full turn produces discomfort. Even a small rotation, five to ten degrees, is effective for the thoracic joints if done slowly and with control.

Exercise 9: Heel Raise Seated

Primary benefits: BETTER BALANCE and STRONGER JOINTS. Activates the calf and ankle muscles while loading the ankle and knee joints, improving the circulation in the lower legs and the joint function that supports rising from a chair.

1. Place both hands lightly on your thighs.

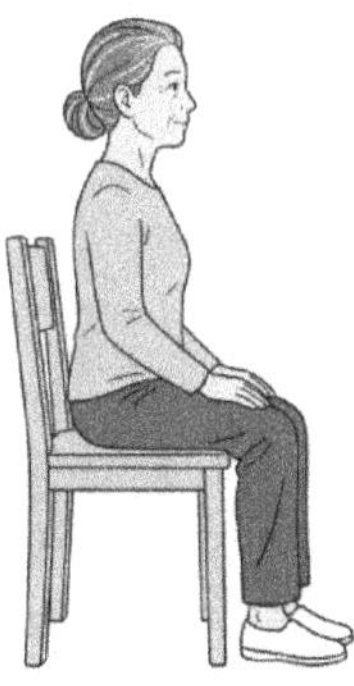

2. Press both toes firmly into the floor and slowly raise both heels off the floor.

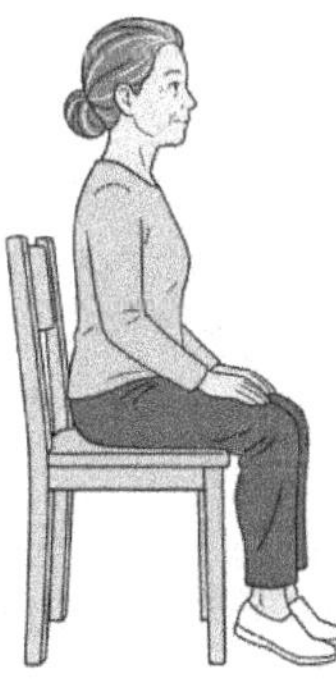

3. Hold the raised position for two seconds.
4. Lower both heels slowly and with control.
5. Next raise both toes off the floor while the heels stay down, flexing the ankles the other way.

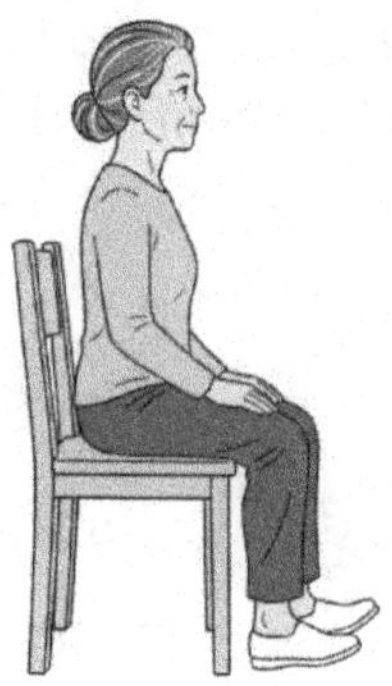

6. Hold for two seconds, then lower the toes.

7. Alternate heel raises and toe raises for ten repetitions of each.

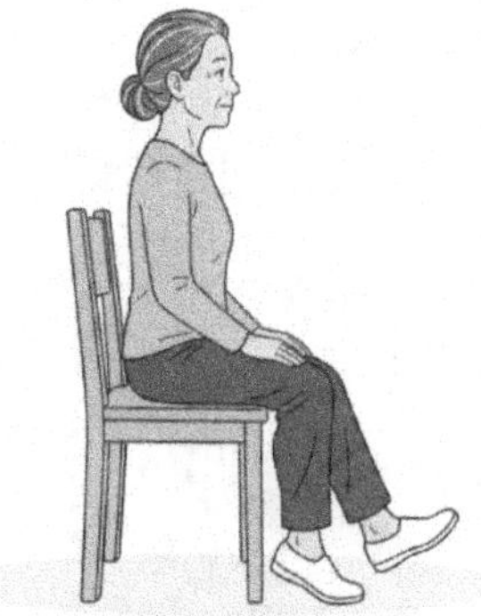

BREATHING: Inhale as you raise. Exhale as you lower.

FEEL IT: A clear engagement in the calf muscles on the heel raise, and a mild engagement in the front of the shin on the toe raise. Both are muscles that support stable walking.

JOINT BENEFIT: Ankle joint loading in both directions, plantar flexion and dorsiflexion, stimulates synovial fluid throughout the ankle capsule and supports the joint's range of motion for walking and standing.

BALANCE TIP: Notice whether the raised-heel position feels equally stable on both sides. An asymmetry often indicates one ankle or calf is weaker. The exercise will address this over time.

EASIER OPTION

Raise heels and toes through a smaller range if the full raise produces calf cramping or ankle discomfort. Half-range repetitions are still effective.

Exercise 10: Still Close

Primary benefit: SHARPER MIND. Closes every session the way Exercise 1 opens it, through breath, stillness, and a return of attention to the body. The closing breath is as important as the opening one.

1. Return to the starting position. Feet flat. Hands on thighs. Spine upright.

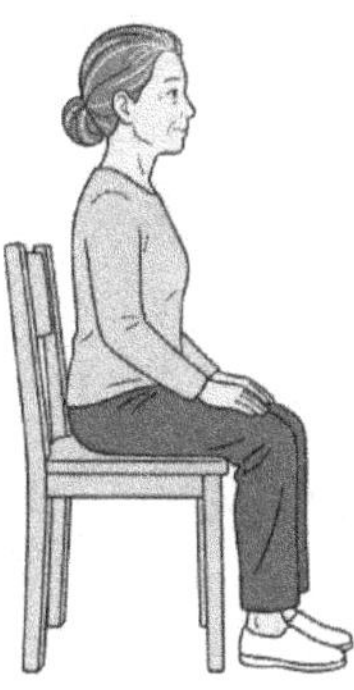

2. Close your eyes or soften your gaze.
3. Inhale slowly for a count of three.
4. Exhale slowly for a count of six. Longer than any other exhale in the session.
5. Repeat three times.
6. After the third exhale, sit quietly for one more breath.
7. Before you stand, notice one specific way the body feels different from the start of the session.

BREATHING: The exhale on the final three breaths should be the longest exhale of the entire session. Take your time with it.

FEEL IT: A settled quality in the chest and shoulders that was not there at the start of the session. This is the physiological result of the work done. Notice it.

JOINT BENEFIT: The extended exhale continues the cortisol reduction of the session into the minutes following, which extends the joint anti-inflammatory window beyond the session itself.

> **EASIER OPTION**
>
> If three long exhales feel like too much, two is enough. The principle is a deliberate slow closing, not a specific count.

Posture Checks: Five Common Mistakes and How to Fix Them

These five errors appear consistently in the early weeks. Each one reduces the benefit of the exercises it affects. Checking for them takes five seconds and is worth doing at the start of each session in Weeks One and Two.

Mistake 1: Leaning Back Into the Chair

Resting the lower or mid-back against the chair back during exercises removes the trunk engagement that makes the exercises work. The chair back is for rest between sessions, not for support during them.

The fix: sit at the front half of the chair seat before each session begins, so there is a gap between your back and the chair back. If you catch yourself drifting backward during a session, return to the front of the seat.

Mistake 2: Shoulders Raised Toward the Ears

Lifting the shoulders toward the ears is the body's automatic tension response to effort, unfamiliar movement, or mild anxiety about performance. It stiffens the neck, compresses the cervical spine, and reduces the shoulder range of motion that the exercises are designed to develop.

The fix: at the start of each exercise, take one breath and on the exhale consciously let the shoulders drop away from the ears. This is an active release, not just a reminder. Check again at the midpoint of the exercise.

Mistake 3: Holding the Breath

Breath-holding during exercises is common in the first week. It happens when the body perceives the movement as demanding enough to trigger a mild stress response. Held breath activates the sympathetic nervous system, which directly undoes the cortisol-reducing effect that is one of the main benefits of the practice.

The fix: if you notice you have been holding your breath, exhale completely first, then resume the breathing pattern. Do not try to catch up to where the count was. Simply restart the breath from the current moment.

Mistake 4: Feet Leaving the Floor

Lifting one or both feet during weight shift or trunk rotation exercises removes the floor contact that provides the balance anchor for those movements. It also reduces the proprioceptive input from the feet that contributes to seated stability.

The fix: before any exercise that involves trunk movement, press both feet firmly and evenly into the floor. Treat the foot contact as an active postural cue, not a passive resting position.

Mistake 5: Moving Too Fast

Rushing through exercises is the most consistent way to reduce their effectiveness. Fast movement produces momentum that carries the joint through its range without the compression-release cycle that delivers the synovial fluid benefit. Fast movement also reduces the proprioceptive training signal, because the joint receptors need sustained, slow stimulation to fire accurately.

The fix: if an exercise starts to feel easy, resist the impulse to speed it up. Instead, slow down and pay closer attention to a specific sensation inside the movement, what the shoulder joint feels like at the top of the arc, or how the weight is distributed across the sitting bone during a shift. The exercise becomes richer when it slows down, not flatter.

A Small Request

If working through this book has done something useful for you even one small thing that shifted, it would mean a great deal to hear about it. Would you be willing to leave a short, honest review on Amazon?

As an independent author, books like this one find their readers through honest reviews not advertising, not algorithms, just one person telling another that something helped them. If the past 4 chapters read so far produced any change you would want someone else to know about, a short review on Amazon is the most direct way to pass that along.

Two minutes. One or two sentences. That is genuinely all it takes, and it matters more than most people realize.

You can leave your review on Amazon by searching the title *Seated Tai Chi for Seniors Over 60 by Liuhe Chen* on Amazon. It takes two minutes, and it matters more than you know.

Chapter 5

Your 28-Day Chair Program

This is the day-by-day program. Each entry tells you exactly what to do, for how long, and what to pay attention to. Read the coaching note before each session. It is short. It matters.

Two things to know before Day 1. First, the rest days are scheduled on specific days for physiological reasons. Do not replace them with makeup sessions. Do not move them. They are placed where the body benefits most from recovery. Second, the exercises reference Chapter Four by name throughout. Having read Chapter Four, you have a picture of each exercise. If you need to review the full instructions during a session, Chapter Four is your reference.

Week 1 – Getting Settled

This week uses three exercises: Settle and Breathe, Arm Float, and Still Close. Sessions are ten minutes. The goal is not performance. The goal is showing up daily, getting the starting position right, and building the breath coordination before adding more exercises. The three exercises you learn this week are the foundation for everything that follows.

> **What You Might Feel This Week**
> • Sessions may feel mentally demanding, particularly in the first two days. This is normal. Learning new movements requires genuine cognitive effort.
> • The starting posture may feel uncomfortable at first, especially in the mid-back. The muscles that support an upright seated position are being asked to work. This improves significantly by Day 5.
> • A quiet settling sensation during Still Close, particularly toward the end of the week. This is the nervous system beginning to recognize and respond to the session pattern.

Your win this week: complete every practice day in full, including the body scan and the closing breath. Consistency over quality.

Day 1 – Your First Session

SESSION AT A GLANCE
Duration: 10 minutes
Exercises: Settle and Breathe, Arm Float, Still Close
Focus: getting the starting position and breath right
Low-energy option: Settle and Breathe only, 5 minutes

Liuhe's Note
Before anything else, complete the three baseline tests from Chapter Three if you have not already done them. Then do the five-minute body scan. Then sit in the starting position for a full minute before Exercise 1 begins. This minute is not wasted time. It is the transition from ordinary sitting into the practice.

NOTICE TODAY
BALANCE: Notice how your weight is distributed across both sitting bones at the start of the session. Which side feels more loaded? That awareness is the beginning of seated balance training.

Day 2 – The Breath Again

SESSION AT A GLANCE
Duration: 10 minutes
Exercises: Settle and Breathe, Arm Float, Still Close
Focus: keeping the exhale longer than the inhale throughout
Low-energy option: Settle and Breathe, three cycles only

Liuhe's Note
Today's focus is exclusively on the breath. During Arm Float, the arms rise on the inhale and lower on the exhale. If the arms and breath fall out of sync, pause, exhale fully, and restart the arm movement from the bottom. The breath is the driver. The arms follow it.

NOTICE TODAY
BALANCE: During Arm Float, notice whether the trunk stays still when the arms rise, or whether there is a slight shift. The trunk steadiness is the balance task inside this exercise.

Day 3 – Rest

REST DAY
No practice session today. Rest is a scheduled part of this program.

Day 4 – Back to the Chair

SESSION AT A GLANCE
Duration: 10 minutes
Exercises: Settle and Breathe, Arm Float, Still Close
Focus: noticing what has settled since Day 2

Liuhe's Note
Most people find that the session following a rest day feels more fluid than the ones before it. If Arm Float feels even slightly easier than on Day 2, that is the consolidation working. Pay attention to it. Recognizing progress makes the next five days more motivated.

NOTICE TODAY
BALANCE: During Arm Float today, can you feel the weight shift very slightly in the sitting bones as the arms rise? That subtle shift is the trunk managing the load of the arms. It is the balance system at work.

Day 5 – Finding the Pace

SESSION AT A GLANCE
Duration: 10 minutes
Exercises: Settle and Breathe, Arm Float, Still Close
Focus: making each movement noticeably slower than feels natural

Liuhe's Note
If the exercises are starting to feel familiar and comfortable, the impulse to speed them up will arrive today. Resist it. Slow down instead. Pay closer attention to the quality of each arm arc, the sensation inside the shoulder joint at the top of the Float. Comfort at the current pace is the signal to deepen the attention, not to move faster.

NOTICE TODAY

BALANCE: Notice whether the weight distribution across both sitting bones is more even today than on Day 1. It may be. Or it may vary. Recording what you notice is more useful than comparing to an expected result.

Day 6 – Rest

REST DAY

No practice session today. Rest is a scheduled part of this program.

Liuhe's Note

The body is adapting. Rest days this early in a program are especially productive because the adaptation processes are running from a larger deficit than they will be in Weeks Three and Four. The joint lubrication and proprioceptive neural changes that the first five sessions initiated are consolidating right now.

Day 7 – End of Week 1

SESSION AT A GLANCE
Duration: 10 minutes
Exercises: Settle and Breathe, Arm Float, Still Close
Focus: your full attention on every step of every exercise

Liuhe's Note

Seven sessions. Complete today's session as if demonstrating the exercises to someone who has never seen them. That quality of demonstrative attention, where you must be clear and deliberate about every movement, is exactly the proprioceptive training intensity the exercises need. Use it on yourself today.

NOTICE TODAY

BALANCE: After Still Close today, sit for one extra breath and notice how the body feels compared to how it felt at the very start of Day 1. Something has changed. Name it.

One week done. The exercises are familiar. The breath is settling into coordination with the movement. The starting posture is becoming more natural. This is exactly where Week Two needs you to be.

A brief note on what you may not have noticed yet: the joint effects of this practice take longer to appear than the neural and breath effects. The cortisol shift that produces the calmer, more settled quality at the end of each session has been building since Day 1. The joint lubrication changes that reduce morning stiffness typically appear at the end of Week Two or the beginning of Week Three. This is not a delay in effectiveness. It is the correct sequence. The nervous system responds first, the joints respond second, and the cognitive clarity improvements tend to follow both. Trust the sequence.

Week 2 – Building Flow

This week adds Shoulder Roll and Open, Seated Weight Shift, and Knee Lift and Lower to the sequence. Sessions run ten to twelve minutes depending on pace. The joint effects of the practice typically become more noticeable in Week Two as the daily synovial fluid circulation accumulates. Many people notice that morning shoulder stiffness begins to ease around Day 10 or 11.

> **What You Might Feel This Week**
> • The three new exercises will feel unfamiliar for the first two or three sessions. By Day 12 the full sequence will feel manageable.
> • Knee Lift and Lower may produce mild hip fatigue in the early sessions of this week. This is the hip flexors working. It resolves within a few days.
> • The Seated Weight Shift may feel unequal between sides. One direction is almost always less stable than the other initially. This asymmetry is what the exercise is designed to address.

Your win this week: complete the full six-exercise sequence at least twice with all exercises feeling connected rather than separate.

The session length this week has increased to ten to twelve minutes. The additional minutes come from the three new exercises, not from doing the existing exercises more slowly. Maintain the same deliberate pace through the original three exercises. The six-exercise sequence should feel like a single continuous piece of work, not six separate tasks with transitions between them. That continuity is what Week Two is building.

Day 8 – Three New Exercises

> **SESSION AT A GLANCE**
> Duration: 10-12 minutes
> Exercises: All six (1-6 from Chapter Four, including three new ones)
> Focus: learning the three new exercises first before running the full sequence
> Low-energy option: Exercises 1, 2, and 10 only

> **Liuhe's Note**
> Do not attempt the full sequence on Day 8. Practice the three new exercises, Shoulder Roll and Open, Seated Weight Shift, and Knee Lift and Lower, separately first. Take two to three minutes with each one. Once each feels familiar on its own, run the full sequence from Exercise 1 to Exercise 6, then close with Exercise 10.

> **NOTICE TODAY**
> JOINTS: During Shoulder Roll and Open, notice whether one shoulder produces more resistance or clicking than the other. That is the shoulder with the greater lubrication deficit. Both will improve.

Day 9 – The Weight Shift

> **SESSION AT A GLANCE**
> Duration: 10-12 minutes
> Exercises: Full sequence, Exercises 1 through 6 plus Still Close
> Focus: the Seated Weight Shift specifically

> **Liuhe's Note**
> The Seated Weight Shift is the exercise that most directly trains the proprioceptive system for seated balance. Today give it extra attention. As you shift right, feel the right sitting bone loading. As you shift left, feel the left. The sensation of weight moving clearly from one side to the other is the training signal this exercise is designed to produce.

> **NOTICE TODAY**
> JOINTS: After the Knee Lift and Lower set today, notice whether the hips feel any different, lighter, less stiff, or different in any way, compared to before the exercise started.

Day 10 – Rest

> **REST DAY**
> No practice session today. Rest is a scheduled part of this program.

> **Liuhe's Note**
> Three new exercises were introduced this week. The brain consolidates new motor patterns during sleep and rest. Tomorrow, Shoulder Roll and Seated Weight Shift will feel more natural than they did on Day 8. That improvement happens today, not during tomorrow's session.

Day 11 – The Sequence Flows

SESSION AT A GLANCE
Duration: 10-12 minutes
Exercises: Full sequence, Exercises 1 through 6 plus Still Close
Focus: the transitions between exercises

Liuhe's Note
Today run the full sequence from Exercise 1 to Exercise 6 without stopping between exercises. The transition from one exercise to the next, coming back to the starting position and moving smoothly into the next one, is its own skill. Notice which transitions feel smooth and which ones feel like you have to pause and remember what comes next.

NOTICE TODAY
JOINTS: During Shoulder Roll and Open today, notice whether the range of motion feels any different from Day 8. Even a very small increase in how far the shoulder rolls before it hits resistance is meaningful progress.

Day 12 – Steadier

SESSION AT A GLANCE
Duration: 10-12 minutes
Exercises: Full sequence
Focus: keeping the trunk completely still during Seated Weight Shift

Liuhe's Note
During today's Seated Weight Shift, focus specifically on keeping the head level and the shoulders horizontal as the weight moves side to side. The trunk tilts, but the head stays level and the shoulders stay parallel to the floor. This distinction requires active trunk control. It is more demanding than it sounds.

NOTICE TODAY
JOINTS: Do you notice a difference in hip stiffness when you first stand up from the chair after today's session compared to a week ago? Record your observation even if the answer is no change yet.

Day 13 – Rest

REST DAY
No practice session today. Rest is a scheduled part of this program.

Day 14 – Halfway Check

SESSION AT A GLANCE
Duration: 10-12 minutes
Exercises: Full sequence
Focus: completing the session fully before the progress check

Liuhe's Note

Complete the full session before you do the progress check. This is important. The check is an
observation of what the practice has built over fourteen days, and it is more accurate if taken
immediately after a full session than before one. Do not try to perform differently because of
the check. Walk through the exercises exactly as you have been doing them. The check
measures the practice, not a performance.

NOTICE TODAY
JOINTS: During today's Knee Lift and Lower, notice whether the hips feel different on lift
number eight compared to lift number one. The warming effect of the repeated exercise on
the synovial fluid is what you are looking for.

PROGRESS CHECK
Two weeks complete. Compare each answer to your Chapter Three baseline numbers.

Seated arm-hold time today (right and left). Compare to Day 1 baseline. BALANCE: a)
Longer b) About the same c) Not yet measured
Morning stiffness rating this week (average). Compare to Day 1 baseline. JOINTS: a Lower
b) About the same c) Variable day to day
Attention drift score today (three-minute count). Compare to Day 1 baseline. MIND: a)
Fewer drifts b) About the same c) Not yet measured
During Seated Weight Shift, does the shift feel more equal between sides than on Day 8?
BALANCE: a) More equal b) About the same c) One side still noticeably weaker
Is morning shoulder stiffness different from Week One? JOINTS: a) Easing sooner b)
About the same c) Still observing

Week Three adds four more exercises and a full twelve-minute session. The sequence will feel
demanding for the first two or three days. By Day 18 it will be flowing. Stay with it.

Week 3 – Going Deeper

This week introduces the final four exercises: Side Reach, Chest Open and Close, Seated Twist, and Heel Raise Seated. Sessions are twelve minutes. With all ten exercises now in the sequence, the cognitive demand rises significantly. The brain is managing ten motor programs in a single session. This is the week where mental clarity improvements begin to appear in daily life outside the sessions.

What You Might Feel This Week
• The full ten-exercise sequence will feel like a lot to manage simultaneously in the first two sessions. This is the correct response. By Day 18 the sequence will flow.
• Seated Twist may produce an unfamiliar sensation in the mid-back. If it is a stretching or releasing sensation, continue. If it is sharp or specifically painful at a point on the spine, reduce the range and consult your doctor.
• Some people report noticeably clearer thinking during this week, a calmer quality to the day, and easier word retrieval in conversation. These are early signs of the cortisol baseline shifting downward.

Your win this week: complete the full ten-exercise sequence at least once with all ten exercises feeling like parts of a single session, not ten separate things.

Twelve minutes is the maximum session length for this week. The ten exercises at a genuinely slow pace fill that time exactly. If you find yourself finishing in under ten minutes, you are moving too fast. Use the extra time to slow down the exercises that feel rushed, particularly Seated Twist and Heel Raise Seated, which are the newest and the ones most likely to be hurried through while the motor program is still being established.

Day 15 – Four New Exercises

SESSION AT A GLANCE
Duration: 12 minutes
Exercises: All ten (Exercises 1 through 10)
Focus: learning the four new exercises before the full sequence
Low-energy option: Exercises 1 through 6 plus Still Close

Liuhe's Note
As on Day 8, learn the new exercises separately first. Side Reach and Chest Open and Close are straightforward. Seated Twist requires careful attention to keeping the hips still while the upper body rotates. Read the Seated Twist instructions again before attempting it. Take it slowly.

Day 16 – Full Sequence First Time

SESSION AT A GLANCE
Duration: 12 minutes
Exercises: All ten in order
Focus: completing the sequence, not perfecting it

Liuhe's Note
Today run all ten exercises in order for the first time. It will feel imperfect. Some transitions will be rough. Some exercises will feel forgotten in the middle. All of this is correct for Day 16. The goal is one complete run-through from Exercise 1 to Exercise 10. Finish it. Imperfect completion beats perfect but partial.

NOTICE TODAY
JOINTS: After the Chest Open and Close sequence, notice whether there is any difference in how the upper chest and front-of-shoulder area feels compared to before the exercise. The thoracic opening effect is often perceptible immediately.

Day 17 – Rest

REST DAY
No practice session today. Rest is a scheduled part of this program.

Liuhe's Note
Four new exercises in two days. The motor consolidation required to build all ten exercises into a single fluent sequence takes time and requires rest. Tomorrow you will notice that the sequence feels more manageable than it did on Day 16. The consolidation happens during today's rest.

Day 18 – Settling In

SESSION AT A GLANCE
Duration: 12 minutes
Exercises: All ten in order

Focus: the quality of each exercise rather than the memory of the sequence

Liuhe's Note

After yesterday's rest, the sequence should feel slightly more available. Today shift the attention from remembering what comes next toward paying attention to what each exercise feels like from inside. Settle into the Arm Float. Feel the thoracic twist of Seated Twist. Notice the calf engagement in Heel Raise Seated. The exercises are the same. The quality of attention is what changes.

NOTICE TODAY

MIND: After Still Close today, sit for one extra breath and notice the quality of your thinking. Is there any difference in mental clarity or calmness compared to before the session began? Even a small shift is worth noting.

Day 19 – The Twist

SESSION AT A GLANCE

Duration: 12 minutes
Exercises: All ten in order
Focus: Seated Twist specifically

Liuhe's Note

Seated Twist is the exercise that most directly addresses the thoracic joint stiffness that prolonged sitting creates. Today give it the full slow attention it needs. Rotate only as far as is comfortable without the hips following. Hold the rotated position for a full three-second count on each side. Do not rush through it to get to the next exercise.

NOTICE TODAY

MIND: During Seated Twist today, keeping the hips still while the upper body rotates requires sustained attention and coordination. Notice whether the cognitive demand of this exercise is different from the others in the sequence.

Day 20 – Rest

REST DAY

No practice session today. Rest is a scheduled part of this program.

Liuhe's Note

The second rest day of Week Three. The thoracic joint mobilization that the Seated Twist and Chest Open and Close exercises have been providing this week consolidates during rest.

Morning mid-back stiffness typically improves most noticeably in the second half of Week Three and into Week Four. If you have not noticed this change yet, this rest day is where much of it is being prepared.

Day 21 – Three-Week Check

SESSION AT A GLANCE
Duration: 12 minutes
Exercises: All ten in order
Focus: running the full sequence with full attention from start to finish

Liuhe's Note
Complete today's session fully before the progress check. Walk through all ten exercises with the quality of attention you would give them if you knew it was being observed. That quality is the right quality to bring to every session. After Still Close, sit for a full extra minute before opening the progress check. That minute is part of the session.

NOTICE TODAY
MIND: During Settle and Breathe today, count the number of breath cycles that pass before a non-session thought enters your attention. Compare this to the first week. The ability to stay with the breath longer is a measurable clarity improvement.

PROGRESS CHECK
Three weeks complete. Compare to your Chapter Three baselines and to your Day 14 check.

Seated arm-hold time today. BALANCE: Right (sec.) Left (sec.) a) Better b) Same c) Variable compared to Day 14.
Morning stiffness this week. JOINTS: a) Further reduced from Day 14 b) Same as Day 14 c) Variable
Attention drift score today. MIND: a) Fewer drifts than Day 14 b) Similar c) Not yet measured
Does the Seated Twist produce a noticeable mid-back releasing sensation? JOINTS: a) Yes, clearly b) Mild c) Not yet
Have you noticed any clarity or attention changes in daily life outside the sessions this week? MIND: a) Yes   b) Not yet
Which exercise in the sequence in ALL THREE benefits above feels most natural today?

Week Four adds no new exercises. It extends the session slightly and asks you to bring the quality of attention you have built over three weeks to a program that is now fully yours. The work is the same. What changes is how well you know it.

Week 4 – Making It Yours

No new exercises this week. The same ten exercises, in the same sequence, for twelve minutes daily. Week Four is about depth, not breadth. You know the exercises well enough now that the attention can go inside them rather than onto them. This is where the three benefits tend to consolidate into something that feels reliably different from how the body felt before Day 1.

What You Might Feel This Week

• The full sequence will flow more naturally this week than it did at any point in the program. Familiar sequences require less conscious management, freeing attention for the proprioceptive and breath work the exercises are designed to produce.

• Some people notice changes in how they feel when rising from a chair, reaching for objects, or sitting in moving vehicles during this week. These are the daily life transfers of what the practice has been building.

• The closing session on Day 28 will feel different from Day 1 in ways that are worth sitting with for a moment after Still Close.

Your win this week: complete every session including the full body scan and closing breath. Leave no session unfinished.

Week Four asks for the same twelve minutes as Week Three but delivers a noticeably different experience. The difference is not in the exercises. It is in the familiarity with them. An exercise you are learning asks for your attention at the level of remembering the steps. An exercise you know asks for your attention at the level of what the joint feels like, what the breath is doing, whether the balance cue is being honored. Week Four is the week for that second and deeper level of attention. It is also the week where the daily life transfers become most noticeable, because the proprioceptive and joint changes have had four weeks to accumulate.

Day 22 – Full Attention

SESSION AT A GLANCE
Duration: 12 minutes
Exercises: All ten in order
Focus: bringing full attention to each exercise rather than tracking what comes next

Liuhe's Note
The sequence is familiar enough now that you do not need to track what comes next. Use that freed attention. During Arm Float, feel the weight distribution across both sitting bones

shifting as the arms rise. During Seated Twist, feel the thoracic vertebrae rotating individually. The sequence is the vehicle. The sensation is the destination.

NOTICE TODAY
ALL THREE: Today notice one thing about each benefit area during the session: one thing about balance, one about joints, one about your mental clarity or calmness. Write them down after Still Close.

Day 23 – The Joints Today

SESSION AT A GLANCE
Duration: 12 minutes
Exercises: All ten in order
Focus: the joint sensation in every exercise

Liuhe's Note
Today make joints the focus. In every exercise, pay specific attention to what the relevant joint feels like during the movement. The shoulder during Arm Float. The hip during Knee Lift. The ankle during Heel Raise Seated. The thoracic spine during Seated Twist. Four weeks of synovial work has been building something specific in each of those joints. Today's session is a chance to take stock of it.

NOTICE TODAY
JOINTS: By the end of today's session, which joint feels most noticeably different from how it felt at the start of the program? Name it. Describe the difference as specifically as you can.

Day 24 – Rest

REST DAY
No practice session today. Rest is a scheduled part of this program.

Liuhe's Note
The session on Day 23 asked a lot of each joint in the sequence. Today those joints consolidate the progress that the last three weeks have built. A rest day in Week Four carries more accumulated change than a rest day in Week One. The body has more to consolidate.

Day 25 – Balance Day

SESSION AT A GLANCE
Duration: 12 minutes
Exercises: All ten in order
Focus: every seated balance cue in every exercise

Liuhe's Note
Today make balance the focus. During every exercise, return to the balance tip from Chapter Four. Keep both feet anchored in Seated Twist. Keep the trunk vertical in Side Reach. Feel the weight shift clearly in Seated Weight Shift. Three weeks of proprioceptive training has sharpened these responses. Today is the session to notice how much.

NOTICE TODAY
BALANCE: Repeat the seated arm-hold test from Chapter Three at the end of today's session. Hold each arm out at shoulder height and count how long it holds level. Compare to your Day 1 baseline.

Day 26 – Mind Day

SESSION AT A GLANCE
Duration: 12 minutes
Exercises: All ten in order
Focus: the mental clarity and attention quality of the session itself

Liuhe's Note
Today make the mind the focus. Start with three breath cycles in Settle and Breathe and notice how long it takes before a non-session thought arrives. Move through the sequence tracking how much of the attention stays with the exercises. During Still Close, notice the quality of thinking after the session compared to before it. The clarity is the practice working. Name it.

NOTICE TODAY
MIND: After Still Close, rate the quality of your thinking on a scale of one to five. One is foggy and distracted. Five is clear and present. Compare to how you would have rated it before Day 1.

Day 27 – Rest

REST DAY
No practice session today. Rest is a scheduled part of this program.

Liuhe's Note

Day 28 – Your Final Session

SESSION AT A GLANCE
Duration: 12 minutes
Exercises: All ten in order
Focus: the complete session with full attention, then the final progress check

Liuhe's Note
This is the last session of the program. Walk through all ten exercises with full attention from start to finish. Do not rush through familiar exercises. Give each one the same quality of attention you gave Exercise 1 on Day 1. After Still Close, remain seated for an extra two minutes. Notice the body. Notice the thinking. Notice the sitting bones against the chair. Let the session fully land before you reach for the progress check.

NOTICE TODAY
ALL THREE: In the final minute of seated stillness after the session, name one specific change in each of the three benefit areas. One for balance. One for joints. One for mind. Be specific. These are the results of four weeks of work.

PROGRESS CHECK
Day 28. The final check. Return to your Chapter Three baseline numbers and your Day 14 and Day 21 check records.

Seated arm-hold today: Right (sec.) Left (sec.) Change from Day 1 baseline.
BALANCE: a) Significant improvement b) Moderate improvement c) Small improvement
d) No change
Morning stiffness rating this week. Change from Day 1 baseline. JOINTS: a) Clearly lower
b) Somewhat lower c) No change
Attention drift score today. Change from Day 1 baseline. MIND: a) Fewer drifts b) About
the same c) Not measured
Name the exercise where you feel the most proprioceptive awareness compared to Day 1.
BALANCE:
Name the joint that feels most improved by the program. JOINTS:
Name one specific change in daily life that you attribute to this practice. ALL THREE
exercises:

Twenty-eight days. The practice is not over. It has a history now, and that history is the foundation for what comes next. The body that completes Day 28 is not the same body that started Day 1. The balance has shifted. The joints have been moved in ways they were not being moved before. The cortisol has been lower, daily, for four weeks. The mind has been asked for ten focused minutes each morning and has delivered them. That is the record. Chapter Eight will help you decide what to do with it.

Chapter 6

Rest, Sleep, and Recovery

The practice days are where the work is done. The rest days and the nights of sleep are where the work lands. This chapter explains what is actually happening during the periods when you are not exercising, and why those periods are as important as the sessions themselves.

Why Rest Days Are Part of the Program

The eight rest days in this program were not placed where they are because it seemed reasonable to give you a day off. They were placed at specific points in the four-week schedule because the biology of physical adaptation requires periods of rest between training stimuli, and because the timing of those rest periods affects how much of the training stimulus can be consolidated before the next session demands more.

Here is what happens during a practice session in simple terms. The slow deliberate movements produce three kinds of stimulus. The joint movements stimulate the synovial membrane to produce more fluid and drive that fluid through the cartilage. The breath coordination activates the parasympathetic nervous system and begins reducing cortisol. The sequential exercise learning builds new motor programs in the brain. All three processes are initiated during the session. None of them are completed during it.

Synovial fluid production increases in response to joint movement, but the full replenishment of the cartilage matrix and the clearance of waste products takes twelve to twenty-four hours. The first few hours of that recovery happen during ordinary rest between sessions. The deepest part of the cartilage repair happens during sleep, specifically during the slow-wave sleep stages of the night when growth hormone is released and tissue repair processes are most active. A rest day gives the joints a full cycle of this repair before asking them to do the work of a session again.

The joint improvements that practitioners notice most clearly on the days after rest days are not coincidences. The Day 4 return after the Day 3 rest typically feels more fluid than Day 3 itself felt. The Day 11 return after the Day 10 rest often shows the first clear proprioceptive improvement of the program. This pattern is consistent and predictable because the biology of the consolidation period is consistent. Understanding it makes the rest days easier to honour, because the improvement on the day after a rest day is both expected and real.

Motor program consolidation follows the same pattern. When a new sequence of movements is learned, the brain begins building the neural connections for the motor program during the session. The actual strengthening of those connections, the process that makes tomorrow's session feel more familiar than today's, happens primarily during sleep. This is why people reliably report that forms feel more natural after a rest day than they did before it. The consolidation happened overnight during the rest.

This is also the reason the program places rest days at the specific points it does rather than simply distributing them evenly through the four weeks. Day 3 comes after two full sessions of learning the first three exercises, when motor consolidation is most needed. Day 6 comes after two more sessions where the pace and posture have been refined. Day 10 arrives after three new exercises were introduced. Day 13 follows the session where the six-exercise sequence was first attempted as a continuous flow. Each rest day is placed after the session that introduced the highest new learning demand, because that is when the consolidation window is most valuable.

The cortisol reduction mechanism also benefits from rest. A single session produces an acute cortisol drop that lasts two to four hours. But the gradual shift in the cortisol baseline that produces sustained improvements in sleep quality, joint inflammation levels, and cognitive clarity, accumulates over weeks of consistent practice. Rest days do not interrupt this accumulation. They are part of the consistent pattern that makes it possible.

This is why the instruction in Chapter Five not to replace rest days with makeup sessions is not bureaucratic caution. It is biology. Doing an extra session on a rest day does not add another day's worth of benefit. It adds one more stimulus before the previous stimulus has been consolidated. The net result is less total benefit than the scheduled program produces, not more. The rest days are designed in. Trust the design.

What Happens When You Stop and Sleep

Sleep is the most productive period across the full twenty-four-hour cycle for the three benefits this program builds. What happens in the body during a well-slept night after a practice day is worth understanding specifically.

In the first hour or two of sleep, the body enters the first slow-wave sleep stage. Blood pressure drops. Heart rate slows. Muscle tension releases. The synovial membranes, freed from the loading demands of the day, resume their fluid production at their highest overnight rate. The cartilage, which was compressed and released during the session's exercises, draws in synovial fluid through the relaxed joint space. The anti-inflammatory processes in the joint tissue become most active during this first slow-wave stage. This is when the morning stiffness of the previous day is most directly reduced.

During REM sleep, typically in the second half of the night, the brain consolidates the motor programs built during the day's session. The hippocampus replays the sequences of the exercises and transfers them into longer-term procedural memory. This is the mechanism behind the feeling of competence that appears after a rest night. The Seated Twist that required active conscious management on Day 15 runs more automatically on Day 16 because the overnight consolidation moved it from effortful working memory into the motor program library.

The glymphatic system, a waste-clearance mechanism in the brain that operates primarily during slow-wave sleep, clears the metabolic byproducts of the day's cognitive work. The prefrontal cortex, which managed the exercise sequences, produced the focused attention, and maintained the breath coordination during the session, begins the following day with its metabolic waste cleared. This overnight clearance is part of why mornings after good sleep tend to feel cognitively sharper than mornings after disrupted sleep.

Cortisol follows a distinctive overnight pattern. Levels are lowest in the early hours of the night and begin rising in the final two hours before waking. This natural morning rise is the cortisol awakening response, a physiological mechanism that prepares the body for the demands of the day. A person who has been practicing the program consistently will have a lower baseline cortisol level overall, which means the morning awakening response starts from a lower floor. The result is a morning that feels less immediately demanding, a smaller gap between sleeping rest and waking readiness. Many practitioners describe this as one of the quieter but most welcome changes from the program.

Habits That Help Your Practice

The quality of sleep you get after each practice day directly affects how much of that day's work consolidates. These four evening habits support that quality. Each takes less than five minutes.

The first is the end-of-day joint release. In the ten minutes before bed, while seated or lying down, perform gentle ankle circles in both directions, slowly roll both shoulders backward three times, and place both hands on your knees and gently bend each knee a small amount while seated at the edge of the bed. These micro-movements stimulate a small final pulse of synovial fluid through the three main joint areas the program works on. The joints begin the night in a more lubricated, less inflammatory state than they would without this brief sequence.

The second is the three-breath close. Sitting on the edge of the bed before lying down, complete three slow breath cycles using the same pattern as the Still Close exercise from the program: inhale for three counts, exhale for six. This brief parasympathetic activation reduces the cortisol level entering sleep and supports the transition into slow-wave sleep. It takes under two minutes.

The third is reducing screen brightness in the hour before bed. The blue-spectrum light from screens delays the onset of melatonin and pushes the sleep onset later, shortening the window for slow-wave sleep. Dimming the screen or switching to a warm light mode in the final hour before bed is a small adjustment that produces a meaningful improvement in sleep architecture over time.

The fourth is avoiding a significant meal in the two hours before sleep. Digestion during sleep competes with the repair and consolidation processes that the program depends on. A light snack if hunger is an issue is fine. A full meal within two hours of sleep reduces the depth of slow-wave sleep and slows the overnight processes that the practice days have initiated.

None of these habits requires discipline or sacrifice. They are small adjustments that create better conditions for what the program is already trying to do. Consistent evening habits compound with the daily practice to produce results that the practice alone, without adequate sleep recovery, cannot fully deliver.

Resting More and Pushing Gently

The program provides a clear schedule of rest and practice. But bodies do not always follow schedules. Two situations arise regularly and are worth addressing directly.

The first is a pain flare. A day when a specific joint is significantly more symptomatic than usual, whether from the exercises themselves, from a separate activity, or from one of the ordinary causes of joint flares like a change in weather or unusual physical demand, requires a response. If the flare is in a joint that a session exercise directly uses, that exercise should be done in its Easier Option form or skipped for that session only. The session itself need not be cancelled. Seated Weight Shift can run without full Knee Lift range. Arm Float can run without the Shoulder Roll. The session structure holds even when individual exercises need modification.

If a pain flare affects multiple joints simultaneously or is severe enough to make the starting position uncomfortable, take an unscheduled rest day. One additional rest day in the program is not a significant disruption. Two consecutive unscheduled rest days, which is sometimes necessary after an illness or a significant physical demand, means returning to the program at the beginning of the current week rather than picking up where you left off. The re-entry at the beginning of a familiar week, rather than at a point in the middle of it, is almost always faster than it sounds.

The second situation is a period of low energy that is not joint-specific. Fatigue, disrupted sleep, emotional stress, or the general low-capacity days that occur for older adults more frequently than most exercise programs acknowledge. The Easier Option within the program's session structure was designed for exactly these days. A session done at reduced range with the same breath coordination and the same deliberate pace delivers the cortisol reduction and the joint fluid benefits of a full session. It does not deliver the full proprioceptive training stimulus, but it preserves the daily habit, which is the most important variable in the program's long-term effectiveness. A reduced session done consistently beats a perfect session done only when conditions are ideal.

There is also a third situation that deserves a direct response: the week when practice simply did not happen. An illness, a family emergency, a significant disruption to the routine that meant several sessions were missed. The appropriate response is not to treat the missed days as lost and the program as failed. It is to re-enter at the beginning of the current week rather than at the current day. A partial week does not have the consolidation structure of a full one. Beginning the week again means completing the intended rest and practice pattern in the correct sequence. This adds days to the program. It does not restart the benefits that were built before the disruption.

Chapter 7

Carrying the Benefits Into Daily Life

The ten minutes a day of this program builds specific capacities in the body and mind. This chapter describes how those capacities show up in the other twenty-three hours and fifty minutes of each day. This chapter is about how to recognize those capacities when they show up and how to support them outside the sessions.

From Chair to Floor to Daily Confidence

The balance training in this program targets the upper body proprioceptive system, the trunk, shoulder, and arm receptors that manage seated stability and upper body positioning. As those receptors become more accurate and responsive over the weeks of the program, the changes show up in daily life in specific and recognizable ways.

Reaching across a table for something becomes less effortful. The body no longer needs to brace or anchor visibly before a forward reach because the trunk has developed the stability to manage the reach without extra support. The reach just happens, with less thought about whether it is safe. This is one of the most commonly reported early daily life changes, typically noticeable around Day 18 to 21.

Sitting on moving surfaces becomes less anxiety-producing. The bus seat, the car seat on a winding road, the seat at a table that is slightly uneven, all of these involve the trunk managing small perturbations in real time. The seated weight shift exercises have been specifically training that management. The trunk that has practiced shifting weight deliberately and returning to center for four weeks handles small unplanned shifts with greater ease.

Rising from a chair, one of the most common daily life transitions for this population, changes too. Getting up from a chair requires a forward lean at the hip, followed by a push off the legs. The trunk control that manages that lean is built directly by the exercises in this program, particularly the Seated Weight Shift and the Knee Lift and Lower. People frequently report that rising from a chair feels easier, requiring less push from the arms, after three to four weeks of consistent practice.

The balance confidence that grows from these specific physical improvements is worth naming separately from the physical changes themselves, because it has its own practical consequences. A person who is less cautious about reaching, turning, and moving through their seated life is a person who does more. More reaching, more turning, more participating in whatever they are sitting near. The physical improvement and the confidence improvement reinforce each other, and both expand the person's daily range of comfortable activity.

The social dimension of this confidence change is, for some people, more significant than the physical change itself. Many older adults have quietly narrowed their participation in social activities because certain physical situations felt uncertain: the unfamiliar chair at a gathering, the crowded restaurant seating, the vehicle ride on an uneven road. As seated balance improves, these situations become less of a calculation and more of an ordinary attendance. The practice does not just improve the chair at home. It improves the relationship with every chair everywhere.

Moving Through the Day With Less Pain

The joint improvements from this program are not limited to the ten minutes of the session. The synovial fluid stimulation of the exercises creates a more favorable joint environment that persists for hours after each session ends. Morning stiffness, which is the first measurable change for most practitioners, resolves faster because the joints are starting each day with better overnight repair and better fluid circulation from the previous day's session.

The shoulder improvements tend to be the most immediately practical. Reaching overhead for a cup from a high shelf, putting on a coat, lifting something from a back seat of a car, all involve the shoulder through its superior arc, the range specifically addressed by the Arm Float, Shoulder Roll, and Side Reach exercises. After several weeks of daily circulation through this range, many people report that movements they had been avoiding or modifying because of shoulder discomfort become accessible again.

The hip improvements follow. Rising from sitting, walking after a long period of sitting, negotiating stairs, all depend on hip joint mobility and the muscular function that surrounds the hip. The Knee Lift and Lower and the Seated Weight Shift exercises both contribute to hip joint health in the flexion and lateral loading ranges that are most affected by prolonged sitting. People typically notice hip improvements slightly later than shoulder improvements, usually in Weeks Three and Four.

The thoracic spine, the mid-back region between the shoulder blades, responds to the Seated Twist and Chest Open and Close exercises. Turning to look behind you, twisting to retrieve something from a different direction, the movements that require spinal rotation, become freer as the thoracic facet joints receive the rotational stimulation the program provides daily. Many people also notice a reduction in the general mid-back achiness that prolonged sitting creates, as the thoracic exercises directly address the compressed posture that generates that ache.

One practical tip for supporting the joint improvements throughout the day: take brief movement breaks every forty-five to sixty minutes when sitting for extended periods. These need not be formal exercises. Standing, walking to the kitchen, doing three slow shoulder rolls, raising and lowering the heels while seated. Two minutes of movement every hour maintains synovial fluid circulation through the joints that the program is conditioning. The daily practice sets the foundation. The hourly movement breaks help sustain it across the full day.

A note on pain during daily life activities. As joint mobility improves through the program, some people notice that they instinctively begin attempting movements they had been avoiding, overhead reaches, fuller spinal rotations, longer walks. This is a positive sign and should generally be encouraged with gradual expansion rather than avoided. The joint health improvements are real. Testing them gradually in daily life contexts, rather than returning abruptly to full pre-pain activity, allows the body to confirm the improvement at each step. Gradual expansion of daily activity range compounds with the program's benefits to produce changes well beyond what the sessions alone provide.

Staying Clear and Present Between Sessions

The mental clarity improvements from this program operate through two overlapping mechanisms that produce their effects at different times of day and in different ways. Understanding both helps you notice them when they arrive and helps you support them.

The first mechanism is the acute cortisol reduction of each session. For two to four hours after each practice, the cortisol level is measurably lower than it would otherwise be. The prefrontal cortex, operating in this lower-cortisol environment, performs better. Attention is more available, word retrieval is faster, complex thoughts are easier to form and hold. Many practitioners notice this post-session clarity peak, a window of particularly clear thinking in the morning hours immediately following practice. This window is real and it is physiological. It can be used intentionally: if there are tasks requiring concentrated thought or clear communication, the two hours following the morning practice is a reliably better cognitive window than the same period without a session.

The second mechanism is the cumulative baseline shift. Over weeks of daily practice, the resting cortisol baseline gradually lowers. This does not produce an acute peak of clarity. It produces a general raising of the floor: mornings that feel more manageable, afternoons with less of the fog that accumulated in earlier months, thinking that is more reliably available throughout the day rather than only in good spells. This baseline shift is less dramatic than the acute post-session window, but it is more durable and more broadly beneficial across the full day.

Sleep quality is the third contributor to sustained daily clarity, and it operates through both mechanisms. Better sleep produces better overnight brain clearance, which produces clearer mornings independent of the session. And the cortisol reduction of the daily practice is one of the most consistent contributors to improved sleep architecture. The practice, the sleep, and the daytime clarity are a triangle: each one supports the other two.

5 Habits That Help What the Practice Builds

These five habits take less than two minutes each. They are not additional exercises. They are daily life movements that reinforce the same systems the practice sessions train, so that the benefits of the sessions extend across the full day rather than fading between them.

First: the seated posture reset. Twice a day, when you first sit down in a new chair or surface, take ten seconds to apply the starting position from the program. Feet flat, hip-width. Spine upright from the top of the head. Shoulders dropped away from the ears. One slow breath. This brief posture reset maintains the postural muscle tone that the program is building and prevents the gradual drift back into rounded posture that happens when the reset is not practiced.

Second: the morning ankle and shoulder warm-up. Before getting out of bed, while still seated on the edge of the mattress, circle both ankles slowly five times in each direction and roll both shoulders backward three times. This thirty-second morning sequence initiates synovial fluid circulation in the ankle and shoulder joints before they are loaded by the day's activities. It does not replace the session. It is a brief preparatory sequence that reduces the discomfort of the first steps and reaches of each morning.

Third: the deliberate breath during daily tasks. When doing something that does not require active thinking, washing dishes, folding clothes, sitting in a waiting room, practice three cycles of the session breath: in for three counts, out for five. This brief practice maintains the parasympathetic activation that the session produces and extends the cortisol-lowering effect into more hours of the day.

Fourth: the standing transition. Every time you stand up from a chair, pause for one second at the top of the stand before moving. Stand fully upright, let the balance settle, then walk. This one-second pause is a micro-proprioceptive training moment. The brief standing balance challenge reinforces the trunk and hip stability that the program develops and creates a small daily life transfer of the seated balance training into a standing context.

Fifth: the evening joint check. As part of the pre-sleep routine described in Chapter Six, take thirty seconds to notice which joints feel different from this morning. Not a medical assessment. A simple check-in: are the shoulders more mobile than this morning? Is the mid-back easier to turn? Has any stiffness that was present at the day's start resolved? This noticing habit trains the proprioceptive awareness that the program builds and makes the progress checks at Days 14, 21, and 28 more meaningful because you have been observing your body consistently rather than only on check days.

Chapter 8

What Comes After Day 28

The formal program has ended. The practice has not. This chapter helps you read the Day 28 records honestly, understand what they mean, and make a clear decision about what the next chapter of the practice looks like.

Reading Your Progress Honestly

The Day 28 progress check produced numbers and observations. Before deciding anything about what to do next, look at those records carefully and honestly. There are three ways to read them and each points toward a different response.

Clear improvement across all three benefit areas, better arm-hold times, lower stiffness ratings, fewer attention drifts, and at least one specific named daily life change, is the best possible outcome. It is also quite common in people who completed the program consistently. If this is your result, the most important decision you face is not what to do next. It is what to protect. The improvements you have recorded are the product of four weeks of daily practice. They are not permanent without continued practice. They will persist and build as long as the practice continues, and they will gradually diminish if the practice stops. The decision to continue is both obvious and necessary. The decision about how to continue is the one this chapter addresses.

Partial improvement, clear change in one or two of the three benefit areas but not all three, is the most common outcome. It is not a failure. The three benefits develop on different timelines, and four weeks is the beginning of the process, not its completion. A person who shows clear joint improvements but has not yet noticed cognitive changes has not done anything wrong. The cortisol mechanism takes longer in some people than others to produce a measurable baseline shift. A second program run will almost always produce improvements in the areas that did not yet show clearly in the first.

No measurable change across all three areas, despite completing the program fully, is the least common outcome and the one that warrants the most careful honest reflection. If the

Day 28 numbers are essentially the same as the Day 1 baselines across all three areas, there are three possible explanations. The sessions may have been done at too fast a pace to produce the proprioceptive and synovial fluid stimulation the exercises are designed to provide. The sleep quality may have been insufficient to allow the overnight consolidation that completes what the sessions initiate. Or the specific condition affecting the most symptomatic joints may require a level of clinical support that a home exercise program cannot provide on its own. The next section addresses this last possibility directly.

Choosing What to Do Next

There are three sensible options after Day 28.

Repeating the program is the option that most people who have benefited from the first run will find produces the most value. The second run of a familiar program is a qualitatively different experience from the first. The exercises are known. The motor programs are built. The attention that was consumed by remembering what came next is now available to go inside the exercises, to notice what the shoulder joint feels like at the top of the Arm Float arc, to track the weight shift through the sitting bones with real precision, to stay with the breath coordination through the full session without it falling out of rhythm. Everything the first run built becomes the foundation from which the second run develops.

Continuing daily practice using the exercises freely, without following the program's daily structure, is the option for people who have integrated the exercises well enough that they no longer need the session-by-session guidance of Chapter Five. This means maintaining a daily ten-to-twelve-minute practice using any combination of the ten exercises, guided by what the body scan at the start of each session suggests would be most useful that day. The body scan from Chapter Three remains the starting point for every session. The Still Close from Exercise 10 remains the ending point. The middle can be shaped by what the joints and attention are asking for on any given morning.

Extending the practice by adding new exercises or exploring a more formal Tai Chi practice under the guidance of an instructor or a dedicated standing Tai Chi program is the option for people who want to develop beyond what this book provides. The seated Tai Chi principles in this program, slow deliberate movement, breath coordination, proprioceptive attention, transfer directly into any Tai Chi-based practice. The foundation this program built is genuine. It is a real starting point, not a preparatory exercise.

Whichever option you choose, one structural commitment supports all three: maintaining a daily practice, even at reduced length, rather than moving to an every-other-day or weekly practice. The biology of the three benefits requires daily repetition. Proprioceptive training consolidates most effectively with daily stimulation. Synovial fluid circulation benefits from daily movement. Cortisol baseline reduction depends on consistent daily parasympathetic activation. Any of the three options above delivers its full potential only with daily practice behind it.

The program provides twenty-eight days of clear structure. Beyond Day 28, the structure belongs to you. The body scan before every session, the Settle and Breathe to open, the Still Close to end. These three bookends are all you need to build a daily practice around whatever exercises serve the body best on any given morning. They work on the difficult days too, when time is short. A session that opens and closes properly, even if only two or three exercises fill the middle, is a complete practice day. The habit holds. The benefits continue.

Next Step When Joints Still Hurt

If joint pain in a specific area has not improved after four weeks of this program, or has actually worsened, there are some practical distinctions to make before deciding what to do.

Pain that increased gradually over the course of the program, particularly in a joint that was already significantly symptomatic before Day 1, is the most likely indicator that the exercise is reaching that joint but the structural condition of the joint may be more advanced than gentle movement alone can address. This does not mean the program was wrong to attempt. Gentle movement is appropriate and beneficial for most degrees of joint disease. It means that clinical assessment and possibly clinical management alongside the exercise program is the appropriate next step. A physiotherapist or rheumatologist can advise on whether the exercise should be modified, supplemented with other treatments, or temporarily reduced.

Pain that appeared suddenly during a specific exercise after a period of comfortable practice usually indicates a technique issue rather than a structural one. Returning to Chapter Four and reading the exercise description again carefully, particularly the JOINT BENEFIT cue and the EASIER OPTION, often identifies the element that needs adjustment. The most common technique problems that produce acute exercise-related pain are range that exceeds what the joint is ready for, speed that is faster than slow-and-deliberate, and starting position that places the joint in a compressed or rotated state before the exercise begins. Address the technique before concluding that the exercise itself is the problem.

Pain that has been present throughout the program at a consistent level, neither improving nor worsening, in a joint that is not a primary target of the exercises, is the most neutral finding. It suggests neither that the program is causing harm nor that it is addressing this particular joint. It simply means this particular joint has a separate issue that this program was not designed to reach. Continuing the program for the benefits it does provide while managing this specific joint separately through its own appropriate treatment is the practical response.

Keeping the Practice Going for Good

The single most reliable predictor of whether a daily practice persists beyond the end of its formal program is whether it is embedded in a fixed routine rather than depending on daily motivation. Motivation varies. A fixed morning routine does not.

The structure that keeps this practice going is simple: same time, same chair, same body scan before the first exercise. When those three anchors are consistent, the practice occurs because the environment cues it, not because of a deliberate decision each morning. The deliberate decision was made once, at the start. The environment does the rest.

When the routine is disrupted, as it will be, travel, illness, family demands, the response that maintains the most ground is a shortened session rather than a missed one. Three minutes of Settle and Breathe, Arm Float, and Still Close, done on a difficult morning in an unfamiliar chair, preserves the daily habit. The habit is worth more than the session. A session missed breaks the chain. A reduced session does not.

The practice belongs to you now. The chair is the tool. The ten exercises are the method. The three benefits are the direction. Keep sitting down and attending to how the body moves. Everything this program built continues as long as you do.

Did You Find This Book Quite Helpful?

If it did, then that's worth something and deserves a place on Amazon.

Leaving a review takes two minutes and nothing else. For a book like this one, written without a publisher's marketing team or advertising spend, that two minutes is how it finds its next reader. It is how someone's daughter spots it while looking for something to give her mother. It is how this work keeps going. Two sentences is all it needs.

Search ***Seated Tai Chi for Seniors Over 60 by Liuhe Chen*** on Amazon. One or two honest sentences is all it takes.

Thank you for reading. It was an honor to take this trip with you.

Conclusion

What Your Body Built in 28 Days

The shoulder joints have been moved through their rotational arc every single day. The cartilage in those joints has received daily nutritional delivery through synovial fluid circulation that it was not receiving before. The morning stiffness that started each day before the program is measurably different from how it starts now. That change is structural. It is built into the joint biology. It persists as long as the practice continues.

The trunk and shoulder proprioceptive receptors have been given specific, daily training through the Seated Weight Shift, Arm Float, and Side Reach exercises. The brain's map of where the upper body is in space is more accurate and more responsive than it was on Day 1. Reaching across a table, turning in a seat, absorbing a small bump or tilt from a moving vehicle, all of these are managed differently now. Not dramatically differently. Reliably differently.

The hip, knee, and ankle joints have received daily loading and unloading through the Knee Lift and Heel Raise exercises. The hip flexors that shortened from prolonged sitting are less tight. The ankle joints have been moved in both directions of their range. The joints that were receiving no deliberate daily movement are no longer neglected.

What Your Mind Built in 28 Days

Cortisol has been lower, every day, for four weeks. The hormonal environment that the prefrontal cortex has been operating in has changed. The thinking that felt foggy, the words that took longer to surface, the attention that drifted more easily than it used to, all of these were partly the results of an elevated cortisol baseline. That baseline is lower now. The change is not dramatic from one day to the next. Across four weeks, it is real.

The three-minute attention test from Chapter Three measures something specific: how often the mind drifts from a deliberate task and needs to be brought back. Four weeks of sessions that required sustained attention to a movement sequence, a breath count, and a proprioceptive sensation simultaneously have trained the focused attention network of the prefrontal cortex. The score on that test on Day 28 is the measurement of that training.

Sleep has improved for most people who complete this program consistently, because the daily cortisol reduction creates better conditions for the slow-wave sleep in which joint repair and motor consolidation happen. Better sleep produces a clearer morning. A clearer morning makes the session easier to sustain. The three benefits and the sleep form a system that, once running, reinforces itself.

A Final Word from the Author

I said at the start that the chair is not a compromise. I want to say it again at the end, with slightly more weight behind it now that you have spent four weeks demonstrating that it is true.

The people who benefit most from this kind of practice are not the ones who came to it in perfect condition. They are the ones who came to it where they were and stayed with it. The person who did every session through stiff mornings and tired days and the occasional feeling that ten minutes seemed pointless. The person who did the Easier Option on hard days and the full version on good ones and kept showing up regardless. That person is where the changes happen. Not in the performance of the exercises but in the decision to return to the chair.

The program is finished. The practice is yours. Come back to the chair tomorrow morning, complete the body scan, and begin with Settle and Breathe. The ten minutes will be different from the very first Day 1 session. The body has changed enough that you will feel it, if you pay attention.

Paying attention is the practice. The chair is just where you sit to do it.

About the Author

Liuhe Chen has practiced Tai Chi for over twenty years. Most of that time has been spent teaching older adults, many of whom had never tried anything like it before and were not sure their bodies were up to it.

Some came after a fall. Some came on doctor's advice. Some came because a friend dragged them along and they ended up staying. Whatever brought them through the door, most of them had one thing in common: they wanted to feel steadier, stronger, and more confident in their own body. That is what Liuhe has spent two decades helping people achieve.

The teaching has always been simple. No complicated moves. No pressure to keep up. Just gentle, steady practice that meets people where they are, whether that means sitting in a chair, moving slowly through joint pain, or starting from scratch after years of little activity. Liuhe has worked with people in their seventies, eighties, and beyond, and has seen again and again that age is not the obstacle most people assume it is.

This book grew out of all those years of working with real people in real situations. It is written for anyone who wants to move better, feel better, and age on their own terms.

Liuhe practices every morning, rain or shine, and still finds something new in it each time.